Grit Pregnancies

HOW TO HAVE A HEALTHY PREGNANCY
AND NORMAL BLOOD SUGARS
WITH TYPE 1 DIABETES

By Allison Herschede, BSN, RN, CDCES

Foreword by Lisa La Nasa

Printed in the United States of America

ISBN: 978-1-7370843-0-3 (paperback)
ISBN: 978-1-7370843-1-0 (ebook)

For information, contact Allison Herschede at Herschede@gmail.com

Editing by Doris J. Dickson.

Cover design by Nicole Buchanan. Layout and typesetting by Jason Frederich.

First Printing, 2021

Note: This book is solely for educational purposes. It is an informative guide about pregnancy and type 1 diabetes. It is not intended as a substitute for the medical advice of physicians. The reader should regularly consult a physician in matters relating to his/her health and particularly with respect to any symptoms that may require diagnosis or medical attention. In no way should this book replace, countermand or conflict with your doctor's advice. All decisions about your pregnancy are between you and your doctor. Although the author and publisher have made every effort to ensure that the information in this book was correct at press time, the author and publisher do not assume and hereby disclaim any liability to any party for any loss, damage, or disruption caused by errors or omissions, whether such errors or omissions result from negligence, accident, or any other cause.

DEDICATIONS

This book is dedicated to the memory of Dr. Lois Jovanovic.
Dr. Jovanovic was a pioneer in the field of type 1 diabetes and pregnancy.
She was rare in her belief in normal blood sugars for pregnant diabetics.

To Matt, Diana, Aidan and Adrian,
thanks for putting up with me writing
this book over the last year and a half.
It took much longer than I thought it would!

Special thanks to Dr. Richard K. Bernstein,
without whom this book would not exist.

Contents

DEDICATIONS.. iii

Foreword xi

Introduction.. 1

   Diabetes in the 1980s.. 2

   The Exchange Diet 3

   Advances 3

   Is a baby possible?.. 5

Chapter 1: High-Risk Pregnancy 8

   So, what are the risks?.. 9

      Miscarriage:... 9

      Birth Defects:.. 9

      Pre-eclampsia/Toxemia: 10

      Progression of Retinopathy: 10

      Progression of CKD:.. 11

      Macrosomia:.. 11

      IUGR (Intrauterine Growth Restriction): 12

      Polyhydramnios:... 12

      Neonatal Hypoglycemia: 12

      Respiratory Distress Syndrome:................................. 12

      Neonatal Jaundice:.. 12

      Stillbirth:... 13

   Anxiety... 13

What is my child's risk of becoming Type 1? 14

Chapter 2: So How Do You Do It? 15

Olivia's Story 15

Carb Counting 16

Bolus Insulin 16

Basal Insulin 17

Types of Basal Insulin 17

Low-Carb 21

Dr. Bernstein 23

So, what do you eat? 23

What if I'm vegetarian or vegan? 26

TypeOneGrit 26

Bolusing Protein? 27

Won't high protein damage my kidneys? 29

Getting the Green Light to Conceive 30

The Rules for the 5 or Less Club 31

Basal Testing 34

Treating Hypoglycemia 34

Four hours after your last bolus: 36

Testing Insulin Sensitivity 37

Chapter 3: PCOS 39

What is PCOS? 39

Chapter 4: The Safety of Low Carb in Pregnancy 41

Doesn't Baby Need Carbs to Grow? 41

What About Ketones? 42

Nutrition 45

Supplements 47

Prenatal vitamin: 47

Vitamin D3: 47

Folate: 48

Magnesium: 48

DHA/EPA: 48

Iron: 49

Chapter 5: The First 4 Weeks 50

Highs-The First Symptom 50

Pregnancy Tests 51

Get on top of it quickly! 51

Insulin Pumps 52

Looping and Pregnancy 56

Pregnancy Targets 58

Making Doctor's Appointments 59

Excerpt from Allison's Pregnancy Blog 60

Chapter 6: Weeks 4-8 61

Insulin Needs; "The Lows" 61

Do Lows Hurt the Baby? 61

Cramping 62

Leukorrhea 62

Excerpt from Allison's Pregnancy Blog 63

Morning Sickness 63

Recipe: Sesame Cheese Crackers 64

Other Symptoms 65

Sweeteners 65

Excerpt from Allison's Pregnancy Blog 67

First OB Appointment 67

Using a Midwife 68

HCG (Human Chorionic Gonadotropin) 68

Miscarriage 69

Chapter 7: Weeks 9-12 70

Symptoms 70

Insulin Needs 70

First Trimester Testing 71

Tests for Mom 71

Excerpt from Allison's Pregnancy Blog 72

"Sneak Peek" Test.. 72

CDE/Dietitian Visit 72

Appetite.. 73

Chapter 8: Weeks 13-16 75

Second Trimester... 75

Insulin Needs 76

Screening and Diagnostic Tests.. 77

Illness.. 78

Chapter 9: Weeks 17-20 79

Increasing Insulin Needs... 79

Dizziness 79

Excerpt from Allison's Pregnancy Blog 80

Leg Cramps... 80

Leg Cramp Remedy Recipe: 80

Anatomy Scan.. 80

Excerpt from Allison's Pregnancy Blog 81

Feeling Movement... 81

Hypoglycemia Unawareness 81

Excerpt from Allison's Pregnancy Blog 82

Chapter 10: Weeks 21-24 82

Insulin Resistance 82

IM Injections.. 83

Excerpt from Allison's Pregnancy Blog 84

Fetal Echo 84

Movement... 84

Alternate Sites 84

Colostrum 84

Excerpt from Allison's Pregnancy Blog 85

Swelling 85

Chapter 11: Weeks 25-28 86

Braxton Hicks Contractions.. 86

Kick Counts 86

Insulin Resistance is Even Worse!...................................... 87

More Tests 87

More Frequent Visits 87

Preterm Labor 87

Premature Baby.. 89

Late Pregnancy Loss 89

    Excerpt from Allison's Pregnancy Blog 92

Chapter 12: Weeks 29-32 92

Third Trimester 92

Estimated Fetal Weight 92

Pre-bolusing 94

Monitoring 94

Weight Gain.. 94

Pumping in the 3rd Trimester.. 95

Pregnancy-Induced Hypertension 95

Preeclampsia 96

Hemolysis, Elevated Liver, Low Platelets (HELLP) Syndrome 96

Pruritic Urticarial Papules and Plaques of Pregnancy (PUPPP)...... 96

Intrahepatic Cholestasis 97

Bladder Pressure 97

Pelvic Pain.. 97

Chapter 13: Weeks 33-36 99

In the Home Stretch 99

The Pump: to Keep or Not? 99

    Excerpt from Allison's Pregnancy Blog 100

Hospital Food 100

Blood Glucose Management 100

I.V. Fluids... 101

Will I be Induced?.. 101

Additional studies and articles 103

What about the risk of stillbirth? 104

Author's Story: Aiden's Birth 106

Will I Need a Cesarean?... 106

Excerpt from Allison's Pregnancy Blog 108

Breech Baby.. 108

VBAC: Vaginal Birth After C-Section.. 108

Monitoring 115

Group B Strep 115

Leaking?.. 115

Decreased Movement 116

Contraction Timer... 116

Chapter 14: Decreasing Insulin Needs...................................... 117

A Whole Chapter? 117

Study 1:... 118

Study 2:... 118

Study 3:... 119

Study 4: 119

Chapter 15: Weeks 37-40 121

Almost There 121

What to Pack 121

Monitoring after 36 Weeks... 122

Sweeping Membranes... 122

Supplements... 122

Author's Story: Aiden's Birth 123

Natural Induction Methods 123

The Big Day... 123

Induction 127

Bishop's Score 127

Prostaglandin Gel 127

Foley Bulb 128

Amniotomy.. 128

Cytotec 128

Pitocin.. 128

Unmedicated Birth/Going into Labor Naturally 128

Home Birth 129

Pain Relief... 130

    I.V. Pain Relief 130

    Transcutaneous Electrical Nerve Stimulation (TENS)............... 130

    Hypnosis 130

    Nitrous Oxide... 131

    Epidural 131

During Labor... 131

Cesarean Section 132

After Delivery 134

Neonatal Hypoglycemia 136

Jaundice.. 136

Chapter 16: Grit Pregnancy Testimonials 138

Success Stories 138

When Things Don't Go as Planned 151

Chapter 17: 40 Weeks and Beyond 154

Going Past Your Due Date.. 154

Postpartum... 154

Postpartum Bleeding 155

Breastfeeding.. 155

Losing the Baby Weight 156

You Can Do This!... 157

Recommended Reading 158

Foreword

Congratulations!!! Let me guess - you're pregnant or planning a pregnancy with type 1 diabetes and you're here looking for support and answers to your many questions. You've come to the right place.

While the media is ablaze with the 'diabetes epidemic' – we face a different reality, the diabetes *EDUCATION* epidemic. We are never adequately taught what to expect during pregnancy with diabetes nor how to effectively control our blood sugar levels in order to avoid common diabetes complications. In fact, diabetes is still considered progressive and debilitating, and diabetes pregnancy is considered high risk because of the standardmanagement protocols. *BUT it doesn't have to be that way.*

We have the power to create health with diabetes and the best possible outcomes for our babies.

As a person with type 1 diabetes for the last 19 years, mother to two girls, ages 13 and 9, and someone who has made diabetes education my life, this book is far overdue. This book made me cry because I wish I would have known this information when I was pregnant with my daughters. This wealth of information and support would have reduced my pregnancy-related stress and worry and would have helped me to be more confident and successful in my T1D management.

Like most women experience, my Endo didn't know pregnancy and my Obstetrician didn't know diabetes. I had so many important questions and no definitive source for answers and support. My medical team was often contradictory in their recommendations and I was alone to figure it out the best I could. I don't want anyone to feel that way.

This book is for every woman who has diabetes and is wondering if - *and how* - she can have a healthy pregnancy, more consistent blood sugar levels, along with less stress and uncertainty.

Allison's informative and straightforward, yet conversational manner is a breath of fresh air to the stuffy, formal medical and pregnancy books that we see so often. We aren't robots, each of our pregnancies is as unique as we are, and Allison understands that fully. She lays the groundwork for WHY diabetic pregnancy is considered high risk - and MUCH more importantly, how to avoid the common issues in the first place.

Truly someone who knows from both personal experience and advanced training, Allison's heart is in helping mothers and mothers-to-be *with diabetes* in their journey of growing, delivering, and nurturing healthy, thriving babies.

Allison Herschede RN, CDCES is the go-to resource for diabetes pregnancy. I'm so incredibly proud of Allison, this book, and all the good she's doing for our community.

Lisa La Nasa
CEO and Founder of diaVerge Diabetes

Introduction

"Grit is passion and perseverance for very long-term goals. Grit is having stamina. Grit is sticking with your future, day-in, day-out. Not just for the week, not just for the month, but for years. And working really hard to make that future a reality. Grit is living life like it's a marathon, not a sprint."

-Dr. Angela Lee Duckworth

I'm Allison. I'm a registered nurse and a diabetes care and education specialist. Yes, that's a mouthful. You might be more familiar with the title, "Certified Diabetes Educator" (CDE), which the title was changed from about a year ago. I'm currently a diabetes coach with diaVerge Diabetes and in addition to coaching diabetics in general, I also offer pregnancy coaching. I'm also a lifelong type 1 diabetic (T1D), diagnosed at 18 months of age. I'm married and have 3 healthy children.

With my first two babies, I had a standard type 1 diabetic pregnancy of counting carbohydrates (hereinafter called carbs) and all that jazz. My pregnancies were healthy and complication free for the most part, but I suffered from *many* low blood sugars, *dangerously* low blood sugars. I took a very large amount of insulin. I also had a very difficult time losing the baby weight. I was lucky. I've seen numerous type 1 pregnancies that did not have the happy endings I did. The really sad part is most of those sad stories were totally avoidable.

With my third child, I was eating low carb, and it was my easiest and smoothest pregnancy. Adrian was my only pregnancy to go to 40 weeks, and I was able to have a vaginal birth after two cesarean sections, which is nearly unheard of in a type 1 diabetic (or in general unfortunately). The pregnancy was complication free, and my baby was completely healthy. He didn't have any of the issues

· · ·

commonly seen in babies of diabetic mothers such as macrosomia (very large baby), hypoglycemia (low blood sugar), respiratory distress, jaundice, etc. Adrian was born completely healthy despite my eating very low carb, which my doctor and CDE had warned against. He is the youngest in his class (totally my fault for inducing before September 1; never induce based on school dates), but almost the tallest, and has been nominated for gifted and talented. He did not need carbs for brain development!

A couple years after Adrian's birth I started following Dr. Richard K. Bernstein's protocols from his book, *Dr.*

Bernstein's Diabetes Solution and was able to, for the most part, normalize my blood sugars. Dr. B's book completely changed my life and my outlook on type 1 diabetes. Type 1 *can* be controlled and as Dr. B says, "diabetics are entitled to normal blood sugars".

I went back to school in 2014 and got my associate degree RN. While working on the floor as a nurse, I was working online on my bachelor's degree and attaining the necessary diabetes self-management education hours required to get my CDE. I received my bachelor's degree in 2018 as well as my CDE (board certification in diabetes as a specialty).

I've been moderating/adminning (is that a word?) diabetes and pregnancy groups for *many* years and have noticed the same questions come up over and over again. I decided to write a book that addresses all these questions, while promoting Dr. Bernstein's protocols. Grit Pregnancies is a Facebook group for diabetics (any kind) who eat low carb and the results this group has seen are in my opinion, unprecedented. Hundreds of women who follow Dr. Bernstein's ways have healthy, full-term pregnancies without complications. Obviously sometimes bad things happen, but they happen to everyone, regardless of diabetes status. When compared to my non-low carb group, the outcomes are *very* different.

This is not a textbook. It is not a book written for medical professionals; it's written for type 1 diabetic women who are pregnant or considering becoming pregnant. There is some textbook data included, but I want this book to come across like I am talking to you personally. I blogged during my low carb pregnancy, so fortunately, I can share my own experience with you throughout this book. Keep in mind that I was not yet following Dr. Bernstein, so I was not getting optimal results. Part of me wishes I could do it again, to do it the right way!

Diabetes in the 1980s

I was diagnosed with type 1 diabetes at the age of 18 months in 1981. It was July and I was super thirsty. I would beg for juice and my mother would give it to me.

One day, I became so thirsty I drank my bathwater. Mom took me to the pediatrician and was told, "it's July, it's hot, of course she's thirsty". Mom wasn't so sure. Her sister had type 1 diabetes, and when she suggested this, the doctor replied, "she's too young for that".

As a certified diabetes educator (CDE), I have seen infants as young as four months being diagnosed with type 1 diabetes. I have heard stories of babies being *born* with T1D, though diabetes diagnosed before the age of six months is typically a form of monogenic diabetes, known as neonatal diabetes. In 1981, this was very unusual, and my pediatrician's office had never diagnosed a child this young with type 1 diabetes before.

Soon after the doctor's visit, I began vomiting. Mom brought me back to the doctor and was told I had the stomach flu and to "give her Gatorade". In the days after that, I lapsed into a coma. My mother rushed me back to the pediatrician's office, and the pediatrician's partner, Dr. Haddock, took me in his arms and ran across the street to the hospital, cursing all the way (he knew immediately what was going on). My blood glucose level came back at greater than 1000 mg/dL (55.5mmol/L).

The Exchange Diet

After being stabilized, I was started on porcine (pork-derived) insulin, urine testing, and a strict no sugar, 1,000 calorie American Diabetes Association (ADA) exchange diet. The exchange diet was a calorie-based diet (1000 calories, 1800 calories etc.) for diabetics which allowed a number of 'exchanges' per day. You had meat exchanges, starch exchanges, fruit exchanges, fat exchanges, and so on. These exchanges were set up to hopefully match your insulin dose (not the other way around like we do today) so if you missed a meal, you went hypoglycemic (low blood sugar). I wasn't allowed things like candy, cake, cookies, or ice-cream. To birthday parties, I brought celery sticks and I gave Trick or Treat candy away or saved it for lows. There are people, especially in other countries where modern insulin is not available, who still use the exchange diet.

Advances

The year I was diagnosed, the first blood glucose meter was approved by the Food and Drug Administration (FDA)and I was lucky enough to receive one, although many people did not get a meter and test strips for several years and continued to test their urine instead.

Around that time the first synthetic insulin known as 'human' insulin called Regular (or R) became available. This replaced the porcine-derived (from pigs) that had been used prior to the development of human insulin. This was lucky for me as I had developed an allergy to porcine insulin.

The first picture shows my first lancing device, known as the "Autolet". It kind of reminds me of a guillotine. It didn't bother me a bit as a child though. The second photo was the first meter I had, the Dextrometer. You had to apply a rather large drop of blood to a strip, wait a period of time, then rinse it off with water (or a wet cotton ball) and the meter would give a result. It was about the size of a rather large book and was pretty heavy.

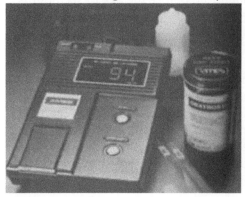 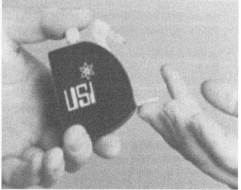

(Photos from "Diabetes, the GlucograF method for normalizing blood sugar", by Richard K. Bernstein, MD)

My parents were told that I would never be able to have children. The doctor stressed that any baby I conceived would be huge, probably deformed and there was a high chance of stillbirth. I would have to spend much of my pregnancy in the hospital, and even if the baby didn't die, it was very possible that I would. This was prior to rapid acting insulin, and all the technology we have today. Pregnancy was very high-risk. Many type 1 women who were diagnosed even a few years before me (and some after) never had children due to this risk.

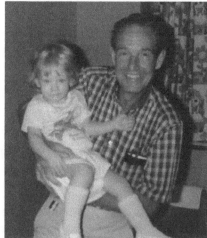

Dr. Haddock holding me after diagnosis, July 1981

As I grew older, several new types of rapid insulin were released. In the late '90s, Humalog (insulin lispro) became available. It was a rapid-acting insulin that was faster and more potent than Regular insulin. Occasionally I was allowed to have something sweet if I ran up and down the stairs 20 times or did 100 sit-ups. This was so difficult to stick to as a teenager, so I rebelled and ate things I knew I shouldn't. I desperately wanted to be like everyone else.

As I departed my teens and entered my 20's, my blood sugars were completely uncontrolled. When I was 19, I went an entire year rarely if ever, testing my blood sugar. I just injected my basal insulin and ate whatever I wanted (usually ramen noodles or rice because I had little money). If I felt low, I ate something sugary. When I did start testing again, I could see that my blood sugars ranged from 40mg/dL (2.2 mmol/L) to 400mg/dL (22 mmol/L) on a daily basis. Sometimes they would even rise well into the 500's and I would go about as normal after popping some Pepto Bismol and taking some insulin. I was called, 'brittle'.

In the year 2000, a first-year family practice resident suggested that I would be a great candidate for an insulin pump. After a few weeks of testing my blood sugar 4x a day (it's hard to imagine I wasn't even doing that!), learning about carbohydrate counting and using a correction factor I was started on a Medtronic 508 insulin pump and it felt like a miracle. Prior to this I was on a standard 'sliding scale', a chart that lists how much insulin should be injected based on the current blood sugar. A sliding scale is completely reactive and does not prevent high blood sugars, it just attempts to correct them.

With the pump I was told I could eat whatever I wanted and use the pump to bolus insulin for it, and I didn't have to take multiple injections every day. It was like I had been let out of prison. I was able to bring my blood sugars down to an a1c of 7 or 8%, which the doctors were much happier with. Hemoglobin A1c is a test that measures what percentage of your red blood cells are 'sticky' with sugar and this percentage gives a rough estimate of the patient's average blood glucose over the prior 3-month period. A non-diabetic has an A1c of less than 5.7% (Dr. Bernstein says a healthy non-diabetic runs around 4.4-4.6%).

Is a baby possible?

Ever since I was a little girl, I wanted to be a mom. I loved playing with my baby dolls and would even pretend to breastfeed them! I planned out names for my future babies. As I moved into my twenties, the movie "Steel Magnolias" resonated in my mind. I didn't want to end up like Shelby and die from having a baby. "Steel Magnolias" is a movie based on a true story about Robert Harling's real-life experience with his sister, Susan Harling Robinson who died from complications as a result of pregnancy with type 1 diabetes. This movie haunted me my whole life. "Oh, you can't have babies. You'll die like that girl in "Steel Magnolias.""

Fast forward to the end of 2003, and it was at about this point that I started thinking about starting a family. I had been with my husband Matt for 3 years, and in this time period, we had not used any birth control. I was worried that I was unable to become pregnant.

I finished my training as a phlebotomist (the person who draws your blood in the hospital or lab) in 2001 and went to work in the hospital. It was there that I saw first-hand all the horrible complications of poorly managed diabetes. It was a very sobering experience. There was one woman I distinctly remember because she was blind from retinopathy (due to high blood sugars, blood vessels in the eyes become leaky, leading to blindness) an amputee, having lost both legs up to the hip, and was on dialysis because her kidneys were no longer able to filter toxins from her blood. For all those things, it was her smell that I will never forget. It was a combination of rotting flesh and this acrid odor of people whose kidneys have failed. We got to talking and I told her that I too was diabetic. Her response was "I'm so sorry". It was at this moment that I truly realized that all those horrible things could in fact, happen to me. Later, after I became an RN, I worked with patients as young as 29 years old, on dialysis, having toes amputated, and requiring a gastric pacemaker (a device that stimulates the stomach to empty) due to gastroparesis. Working as a recovery room RN, I could only give morphine to the suffering patients who had just undergone an amputation. This absolutely killed me, and I knew I had to do something to help prevent these horrible outcomes.

During a routine visit to my endocrinologist in early 2004, it was revealed that my Hemoglobin A1c was 8.7%. "You do not need to get pregnant," the endocrinologist admonished. I told him I was pretty sure I couldn't get pregnant: my husband and I had not used birth control for three years and hadn't become pregnant. I went home and for some reason, this thought stuck in my head, so I took a pregnancy test, and it was positive - faint, but positive!

Matt couldn't see the line on the test, but I could, and I knew I was pregnant. That evening the doctor's nurse phoned and said, "the doctor ordered a beta HCG test (a quantitative blood pregnancy test) and the result is 32 - it looks like you're pregnant".

Pregnant!

My whole world changed after that phone call. My HbA1c was 8.7% and I immediately started to worry that my baby would have birth defects, or I would miscarry, or it would be stillborn. I immediately started testing my blood sugar levels multiple times every day and tried to get them in the optimal range (between 60mg/dL and 120mg/dL) as fast as I could. Usually they were frustratingly high, but I learned that this is one of the first symptoms of pregnancy for many women with type 1 diabetes. Fortunately, my only other symptom was increased levels of fatigue.

By the time I was 6 weeks pregnant, I had my a1c down to 6.3%, (I found out I was pregnant 3 days before my missed period at 3 weeks and 4 days) which was a very rapid drop. I saw an obstetrician at this point and had an early ultrasound due to my being a 'high-risk' pregnancy. There on that screen was my little 'blob', and its heartbeat was steady at 160 beats per minute. At this point, things suddenly began to feel very real -this was no longer something that might happen - it was happening. The obstetrician warned me about all the risks associated with diabetes and pregnancy, such as birth defects, macrosomia (a very large baby) and stillbirth, but he didn't need to bother, because I was already terrified.

Chapter 1: High-Risk Pregnancy

First of all, I want to be very clear on this. The 'risks' associated with diabetes and pregnancy are not due to *diabetes,* they are due to hyperglycemia (high blood-sugar) or from the complications caused by high blood sugar.

Some may think the two are one in the same, but that is not the case. Normal blood sugars are possible, and if your blood sugar is normal, your risk should be the same as a person without diabetes. Now this fact may be questioned, as many studies have shown birth defects and stillbirth even with tight control, but the thing is, we don't agree on the definition of tight control! Most of the studies call, 'tight control' an a1c of less than 6.9% or less than 6.5%. This is not normal blood sugar. To my knowledge there are *no* studies on type 1 diabetic pregnant women with truly normal blood sugars. They don't exist.

An a1c of 6.9% is an estimated average glucose of 168 mg/dL: double normal (according to Dr. Bernstein, a healthy, non-obese, non-diabetic will on average run around 83mg/dL)! A normal blood glucose for a pregnant woman is 60-90mg/dL (3.3-5 mmol/L) fasting and less than 120 mg/dL (6.7mmol/L) post meal. These are targets which are based on the blood sugars of non-diabetic pregnant women. From Dr. Lois Jovanovic's book, *Managing Your Gestational Diabetes*, "For pregnant women who do not have gestational diabetes, blood glucose levels stay within a range of 60 to 120 milligrams per deciliter (mg/dL) (3.3 to 6.7 millimoles per liter (mmol/L). They usually are 60-80 mg/dL (3.3 to 4.4 mmol/L) when measured after a period of fasting (such as first thing in the morning) and less than 120 mg/dL (6.7mmol/L) after eating a meal."

· · ·

These are AACE (American Academy of Clinical Endocrinologists) targets:

Time of check	Blood sugar level
Fasting or before breakfast	60–90 mg/dl
Before meals	60–90 mg/dl
1 hour after meal	100–120 mg/dl

These goals may seem impossible when you first see them, but they aren't! When another life is at stake, your motivation goes into overdrive. Nobody is perfect and we all have bad days, but these goals are attainable, and I'm going to tell you how later on.

So, what are the risks?

All the diabetes and pregnancy books warn you of the complications. They just say these are due to "diabetes" but I'm going to explain WHY we are at risk for these complications.

Miscarriage:

it is considered a miscarriage if you lose your baby before 20 weeks of pregnancy. Miscarriage is pretty common in the general population; in fact, it is said that 1 in 4 pregnancies ends in miscarriage before 12 weeks. 1 to 2 out of 100 pregnancies ends in miscarriage after 12 weeks. The risks are higher in diabetics.

In type 1 diabetic moms, greater than 75% of miscarriages were due to congenital anomalies (birth defects) (Cundy et al., 2007). High fasting blood glucose is also strongly correlated to the levels of hormones mom makes, so if your blood sugars are high, your body may not be making adequate levels of the hormones needed to sustain a pregnancy.

Birth Defects:

Your baby and its organs develop during the first 10 weeks of pregnancy, so if you become pregnant with high blood sugars, birth defects are more likely.

Studies show that babies of moms who are insulin dependent are at a 10-12% risk of birth defects. 3-9% of diabetic pregnancies result in cardiac abnormalities.

Because of this, your doctor will likely have you scheduled for a fetal echocardiogram between 20-26 weeks. Defects of the central nervous system (brain and spinal cord) are 13-20 times more common. Other abnormalities such as cleft palate can also occur. Because of this higher risk, it is super important to have normal blood sugars before and during pregnancy.

"Elevated blood glucose levels at conception and during the early first trimester is associated with increased rates of congenital malformation, of the central nervous system, cardiac, gastrointestinal, and genitourinary tract, are significantly more incident with A1c >7% and the risk is proportional to A1c." (Sugrue & Zera, 2018).

"Data from multiple studies have consistently shown a higher risk of major congenital malformations and miscarriage associated with increasing first trimester glycated hemoglobin values. Although glycated hemoglobin values from different laboratories may not be comparable because of differences in methodology and a lack of standardization among laboratories, a value >1 percent above the upper limit of the normal range is associated with an increased risk of congenital anomalies". (Ecker, Greene, & Barss, 2017)

Pre-eclampsia/Toxemia:

Pre-eclampsia is a condition that only happens during pregnancy. Symptoms include edema (swelling of the extremities and face), high blood-pressure, headache, visual disturbance, and protein in the urine.

The risk of pre-eclampsia is increased two to four-fold in type 1 diabetes. If untreated, it can develop into eclampsia which affects the brain and causes seizures. It is a very dangerous condition. Pre-eclampsia is treated with bedrest and I.V. infusion of magnesium sulfate, but the only cure is delivery of the baby.

"Impaired vascular reactivity in pregnant women with T1DM makes them more susceptible to develop preeclampsia" (Kulshrestha & Agarwal, 2016, para 3).

"The risk of preeclampsia increased significantly with increasing A1C values above optimal levels. Compared to women with A1C <6.1 percent at 26 weeks of gestation, the odds of preeclampsia for women with A1C 6.1 to 6.9 percent, 7.0 to 7.9 percent, and ≥8 percent were 2.1, 3.2, and 3.8, respectively. At 34 weeks of gestation, the odds of preeclampsia with A1C values ≥7.0 percent and ≥8 percent were 3.3 and 8.0, respectively." (Ecker, 2017)

Progression of Retinopathy:

Diabetic retinopathy occurs when high blood sugars cause the blood vessels in the eyes to become leaky and eventually hemorrhage, which can lead to blindness. In moms with diabetic retinopathy,

50-70% have progression of the retinopathy. In most cases the severity of the progression is reduced after the baby is born, but not always.

There is also a known phenomenon where proliferative retinopathy progresses temporarily if blood sugars are normalized rapidly. Dr. Bernstein advises testing IGF-1 levels, and if they are elevated to proceed *slowly* in reducing blood sugar levels. This is definitely something to keep in mind before becoming pregnant if you have proliferative retinopathy. If you do have retinopathy, your eyes will be checked frequently during pregnancy. Many doctors will have a type 1's eyes checked every trimester even if they don't have retinopathy.

Progression of CKD:

If you already suffer from chronic kidney disease, it could worsen as your blood volume goes up and you're filtering more than you were before. This can strain your already weakened kidneys. You'll need to be followed by a nephrologist (which you likely already are) throughout your pregnancy. High blood sugar, as we know, damages the kidneys, so this is another reason it is so important to keep blood sugars normal during this time.

Macrosomia:

Baby is larger than normal (greater than 4000g or 8lb13oz). This is probably the most common issue we see in diabetic pregnancy. When blood sugar is high, that glucose crosses the placenta and raises your baby's blood sugar. In response, the baby makes more insulin to bring it down. Insulin is a fat storing hormone, so this causes your baby to gain weight. Macrosomic babies tend to look like cherubs.

Why is this an issue? Baby could get "stuck" or have shoulder dystocia which can cause brachial plexus injury, a broken collar bone, damage to mom, or even death if the doctor is unable to maneuver the baby out. If you've had a previous c-section, a baby with macrosomia puts you at higher risk of uterine rupture. Many doctors induce labor in diabetic moms routinely due to the risk of macrosomia (among other things), and diabetic moms are more likely to have a c-section because of this.

According to Jovanovic-Peterson and Peterson, "A first-trimester non fasting blood glucose level greater than 120mg/dL increases the risk of macrosomia by 24%. A mean third-trimester non fasting glucose level above 120mg/dL confers with it a 23% risk of macrosomia. Thus, management protocols must include the following: blood glucose monitoring 1 hour after the meal, and (2) therapy designed to keep the blood glucose level below 120mg/dL 1 hour after meals to prevent macrosomia." (Peterson, 1995)

IUGR (Intrauterine Growth Restriction):

Baby isn't growing like it should. This typically occurs in diabetes due to placental dysfunction (the placenta degrades or calcifies, and the baby can't get the nutrients it needs due to high blood sugar). Some studies have shown that low-dose aspirin started at 12 weeks can help prevent this. Diabetic nephropathy or chronic kidney disease tends to go hand in hand with this.

Polyhydramnios:

Too much amniotic fluid. Polyhydramnios occurs in around 1-2% of pregnancies and is more common in moms with diabetes. If your blood sugar is high, your baby's blood sugar may temporarily be high, which can cause more urine output which leads to more amniotic fluid. Also, if your baby is bigger than normal, it's going to have larger urine output. Usually if you have polyhydramnios that is due to diabetes, it is a milder form. If you have polyhydramnios, you have a higher chance of having a c-section due to your baby being in the wrong position or the umbilical cord can prolapse. You will have increased monitoring, and if it is severe, your doctor may decide that some of the fluid needs to be drained to prolong the pregnancy or to relieve discomfort.

Neonatal Hypoglycemia:

When mom's blood sugar is routinely higher than normal, the baby is making extra insulin to compensate. When the umbilical cord is cut, the baby is suddenly cut off from mom's blood supply, and that extra sugar is cut off. The baby is still making extra insulin, so blood sugar drops. Some studies show that if mom's blood sugar is higher than 110mg/dL (6.1mmol/L) when the baby is born, he is more likely to be hypoglycemic. Baby may have to spend some time in the NICU and if blood sugar is very low, may need I.V. glucose.

Respiratory Distress Syndrome:

Due to high blood sugars, the synthesis of surfactant (a substance secreted in the lungs that reduces the surface tension of pulmonary fluids and makes the tissue more elastic so the alveoli in the lungs don't collapse) can be delayed. This is thought to be because of baby making too much insulin, which can interfere with lung development from glucocorticoids. This can cause your baby to have trouble breathing and he may need NICU time. You may be given a steroid shot (Betamethasone) to help mature your baby's lungs.

Neonatal Jaundice:

Due to high blood sugar in mom, and subsequently baby, too much insulin is present in the baby. This extra insulin increases the baby's metabolism, and it consumes more oxygen. Due to this 'relative hypoxemia' your baby produces more erythropoietin (a hormone produced by the kidneys that helps produce red blood cells to carry oxygen) which results in the baby having more red blood cells than normal. The breakdown of the red blood cells after birth results in high levels of bilirubin (an orangish-yellow pigment that is produced by the liver to breakdown red blood cells). This may cause your baby's skin and the whites of its eyes to appear yellow and they may need to spend some time under a special light to bring down the bilirubin levels.

Stillbirth:

If a pregnancy is lost after 20 weeks gestation, it is considered a stillbirth. In years past, diabetes meant a very high risk of stillbirth. Today, with tight control, the risk is close to that of a non-diabetic woman. Recent studies show that there is still a risk, "even with tight control", but their definition of tight control is an hba1c of less than 6.9% which is about double normal blood sugars. Are you noticing a pattern here? HIGH BLOOD SUGARS cause all these complications, not, "diabetes". "When normoglycemia is achieved before pregnancy and moment-to-moment blood glucose control is sustained up to the time of delivery, the infant has the same chance to be normal as those infants born to nondiabetic mothers" (Peterson, 1995)

Anxiety

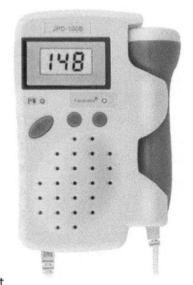

"I feel so overwhelmed like it's consuming me. I have constant fear of going too low & too high... when I have to take a big bolus, I have a panic attack. I've been diabetic for 32 years, but most recently find it hard to deal with".

With all these, "risks" it's easy to be anxious. For the first few weeks I was terrified I would miscarry. Then I was worried about birth defects. Then heart problems. Then stillbirth. Then a c-section. The list goes on.

Honestly, you never stop worrying as a parent, but with type 1, there is even more worry. I was able to buy a home doppler on Amazon that helped calm my mind. A doppler is a device that allows you to hear the baby's heartbeat after around 10 weeks or so. It should not be used as a substitute for medical care and does not guarantee nothing is going on with your baby but hearing that heartbeat can be reassuring. If your gut tells you something is wrong, don't doubt it and get checked.

Any time I was worried, I would listen to my baby's heartbeat and be reassured. The frequent ultrasounds also helped. You can also do first trimester genetic screening to rule out genetic abnormalities which can also put your mind at ease.

While we want our blood sugars as normal as possible, it's important to remember that nobody is perfect, and we are all going to have bad days. You can only do your best. That's all you can do.

When you have a high, and you will, just bring it down as quickly as possible. Dr. Bernstein recommends intramuscular insulin corrections in his book, and I have found these to be quite helpful in bringing down blood sugar quickly.

What is my child's risk of becoming Type 1?

According to Joslin Diabetes Center, "The risk for a child of a parent with type 1 diabetes is lower if it is the mother — rather than the father — who has diabetes. "If the father has it, the risk is about 1 in 10 (10 percent) that his child will develop type 1 diabetes — the same as the risk to a sibling of an affected child, On the other hand, if the mother has type 1 diabetes and is age 25 or younger when the child is born, the risk is reduced to 1 in 25 (4 percent) and if the mother is over age 25, the risk drops to 1 in 100 — virtually the same as the average American" Caucasians tend to be at higher risk that other racial groups. If both partners have type 1, the risk increases to between 1 in 4 and 1 in 10.

Your baby can be tested for the genetic markers for type 1. If you and your baby share the genes known as HLA-DR3 or HLA-DR4, they are at higher risk for developing Type 1.

You can also have your child tested yearly for autoantibodies. Trialnet is a program that does this testing for free in a direct relative who has Type 1 Diabetes, and JDRF is now offering antibody testing for $55. This is subsidized if you qualify.

Chapter 2: So How Do You Do It?

Olivia's Story

I was diagnosed with Type 1 Diabetes at the age of 14. For years I was told that I was doing "very well" managing my disease since my A1C was (slightly) below a 7.0, but I continued to have deep-rooted fears about what my disease meant for adulthood - particularly about the complications that would come with pregnancy. I knew that diabetics had high-risk pregnancies, and deep down, I believed that meant I shouldn't have a baby, or that no one would want me as a wife because I came with the burden of diabetes. Though I always seemed to have my life together, this inner dialogue about my lack of self-worth related to diabetes really affected my ability to thrive. I knew that somehow, I needed to get my A1C below a 6 to have a baby, but I was very healthy, ate well, followed the doctors' orders, and a 6 still seemed so out of reach. When I met my now husband at age 28, I knew that I wanted to have kids with him, and I was determined to do whatever it took to better manage my blood sugars (even though doctors told me I was doing "great" and that I "shouldn't be so hard on yourself").

I had been introduced to Dr. Bernstein about 10 years prior by my best friend's dad. He is type 1, a successful neurosurgeon, had been traveling to New York for in-person appointments with Bernstein himself, and had gotten his sugars so stable it was truly unbelievable compared to my normal. However, my endocrinologist strongly discouraged the Bernstein methods, and scared me out of even trying lower carb. Flash forward to age 28, after being exposed to functional medicine and being more open-minded to trying non-conventional approaches to health. I re-read Bernstein's book, joined the TypeOneGrit Facebook group, and instantly realized that there IS A WAY to have better blood sugars! I was so inspired by the thousands of successful Bernstein followers, so I instantly started low carb.

It only took me 3 months to get my A1C down from a 6.8 to a 5.3. At that first

A1C check post-Bernstein, it was like the weight of the world was lifted off my shoulders! I was so emotional - suddenly, I felt like it was OK for me to have a baby!

3 years later, we were ready to conceive. In those 3 years, I had plenty of time to refine my diet, learn what works best for me, and get my sugars even more stable. I continued seeing a functional medicine practitioner who helped with overall wellness and health. Thanks to the TypeOneGrit Facebook group, I was able to troubleshoot whenever I had issues and learned so many tips/tricks. I joined the Grit Pregnancies Facebook group about 6 months prior to trying to conceive. I had an A1C right around 5 when I got pregnant - with a very small standard deviation of about 20. That roughly means that 95% of the time, my blood sugars were between 80 and 120.

Carb Counting

For my first two pregnancies, I controlled my blood sugar the way I was taught. Count carbs, take insulin based on the estimated carbs, take insulin to correct if too high 2 hours post meal, eat something sugary if low. I was able to keep my a1c in the 5's doing this, but at the expense of *many* low blood sugars and a *lot* of insulin. Fortunately, I had no lasting effects from the lows, but I did have a very scary hypo with my 2nd pregnancy in which the paramedics had to be called. I also gained a lot of weight, which took years to come off. This is the most common method taught and this is how most t1 mommies manage their diabetes.

Bolus Insulin

For those not familiar with carb counting, your doctor or endo will prescribe an insulin to carb ratio, such as 1:15 which is one unit of rapid-acting insulin such as **Humalog or Novolog/Novorapid** for every 15g of carbohydrate consumed. We also have newer ultra-rapid insulins known as **Fiasp and Lyumjev.** So, say you ate for breakfast a bowl of cheerios which is 20g of carb, plus milk that is 6g for half a cup, some fruit that is 20g, and 2 eggs. This is a total of 46g so you would take 3 units, which in theory should mimic the pancreas and keep your blood sugar stable.

Sounds logical when you think about it, but it's not so easy. Exogenous (injected) insulin isn't as fast or as smart as insulin your body makes, and carbohydrate counts on the nutrition label can be off by up to 20%. Insulin absorption can also vary and the higher the dose, the more unpredictable the results.

Your insulin sensitivity or "correction factor" is the amount of insulin you take to correct a high blood sugar, such as 1:50 which would be one unit of rapid-acting insulin for every 50 mg/dL of blood glucose over your target blood sugar. Since the target for post-prandial blood glucose is less than 120mg/dL (6.7mmol/L), anything over 120 would be corrected with insulin. Mealtime insulin and correction insulin is known as bolus insulin.

Types of Bolus Insulin

- **R (regular) Insulin/Actrapid/Humulin S -** short acting insulin
- **Humalog (Insulin Lispro)** - rapid acting insulin
- **Novolog/Novorapid (Insulin Aspart)** - rapid acting insulin
- **Admelog (Biosimilar Insulin Lispro)** - rapid acting insulin
- **Fiasp (Insulin Aspart with Vitamin B3 (niacinamide) and L-arginine** - ultra rapid insulin
- **Lyumjev (Insulin Lispro aabc)** - ultra rapid insulin

Basal Insulin

There is a second type of insulin (or another way rapid-acting can be used) known as *basal* insulin or long-acting insulin. Examples of long-acting insulin are **Tresiba**, **Lantus**, **Levemir**, **NPH** and **Toujeo**. Basal insulin covers the fasting state. The purpose is to keep blood sugar steady throughout the day and does not account for food. Always remember this; basal insulin has *NOTHING* to do with food. You should take it whether you are eating or not. Many healthcare providers don't understand this and hold basal insulin when you aren't eating, which can be very dangerous.

Types of Basal Insulin

- **NPH (Neutral Protamine Hagedorn)/Protamine Zinc/Isophane** - intermediate acting insulin
- **Levemir (Insulin Detemir)** - intermediate to long-acting insulin
- **Lantus (Insulin Glargine)** - long-acting insulin
- **Basaglar (biosimilar Insulin Glargine)** - long-acting insulin
- **Semglee (biosimilar Insulin Glargine)** - long-acting insulin
- **Toujeo (U300 Insulin Glargine)** - long-acting insulin
- **Tresiba (Insulin Degludec)** - long-acting insulin

The only long-acting insulins currently approved for pregnancy are NPH and Levemir, which can be problematic, due to their peaks and duration. NPH is actually an intermediate acting insulin and has a strong peak. Most find they need to take it 2-3 times per day or more. The same is true of Levemir. Many doctors are under the mistaken belief that Levemir is a 24-hour insulin, but it isn't. It can last up to 20 or so hours at a high dose, but its duration is very dependent on your dose. The people who are getting the best results with Levemir tend to take it three times a day. Dr. Bernstein recommends a dose at bedtime, a dose at 4-5am to cover the Dawn Phenomenon, and a morning dose. Others have had success dosing every 8 hours. Work with your doctor or CDE and find out what works best for you.

There have been some studies showing that Lantus (insulin glargine) does not cross the placenta and causes no harm to the fetus, but it has not been officially approved for pregnancy. Anecdotally, many women have had healthy babies using Lantus or Tresiba (insulin degludec). Many doctors will insist on pregnant women only using pregnancy approved insulins and the results can be disastrous if they aren't used correctly. In my opinion, we *know* that high blood sugar is teratogenic (harmful to the fetus), yet the doctors are more worried about *possible* teratogenic insulin, which there is no proof of in the literature. Nobody wants to do studies on a pregnant woman, so the studies are severely lacking.

Dr. Bernstein is not a fan of insulin glargine. Due to its affinity for IGF-1 receptors, in theory, it could increase the risk of cancer.

Always discuss this with your physician and decide what the best method is for you. Rapid-acting insulin can also be used as basal insulin in an insulin pump, which may be preferable during pregnancy.

Insulin: Onset, Peak and Duration

Type	Insulin	Onset	Peak	Duration
Ultra Rapid Analog	Aspart (Fiasp)	2.5 min	60 min	3-5 hr
Rapid Analogs	Aspart (NovoLOG) Lispro HumaLOG/Admelog) Glulisine (Apidra)	5-15 min	30-90 min	<5 hrs
Short	(Regular) HumuLIN R, NovoLIN R, Relion R	30 – 60 min	2-3 hrs	5-8 hrs
Inter-mediate	(NPH) HumuLIN N, NovoLIN N Relion N	2-4 hrs	4-10 hrs	10-16 hrs
Long	Detemir (Levemir) Glargine (Lantus/Basaglar)	3-8 hrs	No peak	6-24 hrs 20-24 hrs
Ultra Long	Deglucec (Tresiba)	1 hour	No peak	<42 hrs

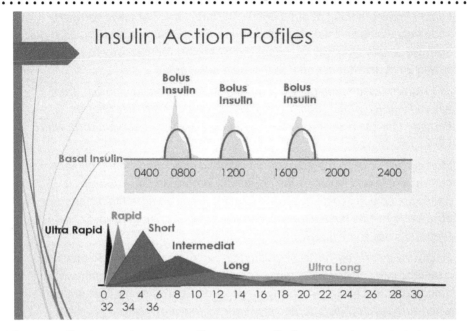

Insulin Action Profiles

Bolus Insulin   Bolus Insulin   Bolus Insulin

Basal Insulin

0400 0800   1200   1600   2000   2400

Ultra Rapid   Rapid   Short

Intermediat

Long   Ultra Long

0 2 4 6 8 10 12 14 16 18 20 22 24 26 28 30
32 34 36

Diabetes Medications; What to Prescribe. Rose M. Flinchum, MSEd., MS, CNS, RN, ACNS-BC, BC-ADM, CDE

There are also mixed insulins on the market that are no longer widely used in the United States, but are still used in other countries. These include Humulin and Novolin 70/30 which is 70% NPH and 30% Regular (also known as Mixtard 30) as well as Humalog mix which is 75% NPH and 25% Humalog and Novolog Mix 70/30 which is 70% NPH and 30% Novolog.

These mixed insulins are for the most part, only used in type 2 diabetics or gestational diabetics. The problem with mixed insulin is that you can't easily adjust the dosage. If you increase one you increase the other and vice-versa.

You can't make a correction for a high blood sugar because you'll also be getting basal insulin. These insulins also require strict mealtimes to avoid hypoglycemia as the food is based on the dose rather than the opposite which we do with basal/bolus insulin.

Sally Ann Clarke recounts her experience using mixed insulin.

It was 2008; I was a triathlete and unexpectedly pregnant. As I was on medications for hypothyroid since 2000, I checked in with my endocrinologist immediately that I found out. He had me do a glucose tolerance test immediately, which I failed at probably around 6 weeks pregnant. He told me gestational diabetes and sent me to a dietitian. I told her I was probably celiac. So she came up with a meal plan that included 7 x 1/2 cup of rice exchanges with 240g of carbs. (1900 cals, 240g carbs, 95g protein, 60g of fat).

I didn't know anything about diabetes at that stage, but I was horrified knowing I would certainly have problems with weight, let alone blood sugar. She also couldn't answer me about adjusting diet for exercise etc. I realized within 24 hours that her approach would not work.

So I started researching on-line. I found articles by Lois Jovanovich, from whom I learned blood sugar control was essential. I also heard of Dr. Bernstein for the first time. I tried to manage with amateur low carb, which worked fairly well.

Starting just prior to the pregnancy I had had abdominal pain. This kept getting worse and worse as the pregnancy progressed. At 3 months it finally got so bad I could not stand straight. I was admitted to hospital for observation while the doctors argued about what to do for about a week as they could not come up with a clear diagnosis.

Finally my elderly obstetrician insisted on exploratory surgery. So they did a laparotomy and appendectomy. The day after surgery I had symptoms of amoebiasis which was eventually diagnosed after calling my obstetrician when surgical staff disregarded my requests for treatment.

Pathology came back as chronic appendicitis. I lost about 8 kg while in the hospital for nearly 3 weeks. It was very lucky my baby survived.

Once I was discharged, I could no longer control blood sugar levels with diet. I was put on mixed insulin twice a day and provided with no training except for a 5-minute instruction on injection. I was given a pamphlet from Eli-Lilly. There seems to be no such profession as a diabetes educator in the Philippines. So, I continued low carb and the insulin with reasonable blood sugar levels. At 8 months pregnant and just before I could no longer travel, I went to China for a tour, with friends. One morning we were packing to leave the hotel. I had taken my insulin but did not get down to breakfast quickly enough (I did not understand the necessity of eating on time with mixed insulin). I woke up in a Chinese Hospital Emergency Room. That was my wakeup call to start learning more, a whole lot more!

I delivered my first born with my A1c at about 5.4! My total daily insulin dose by the time of delivery was about 80 units a day. My daughter weighed 7lbs 3 oz and was healthy. The endocrinologist told me I could stop insulin and no need to test blood sugar anymore; that we would do a glucose tolerance test in 3 to 6 months.

However, by this time I had gotten serious about reading "Diabetes Solution", listened to all the telecasts as well. So I decided to keep testing. Blood sugars were not normal. Not terribly high, but definitely not Bernstein standard acceptable. As I was planning for a second baby as soon as possible I personally decided to keep taking insulin. I changed my insulin from mixed to basal-bolus. Insulin can be bought over the counter here in the Philippines.

I continued low dose basal-bolus insulin for the next 3 years. During this time after failing to get pregnant for six months of trying after menstruation returned, I was doing fertility hormones and IUI to try to get pregnant again: I had several miscarriages. Every time I got pregnant my blood sugar and insulin requirements would immediately rise. Finally in August of 2011, I had another attempt. Within 12 hours of IUI my blood sugars soared. The endocrinologist asked me to do a glucose tolerance test again. Even though I was already taking insulin! I just laughed at him and said, why?

During that pregnancy I increased from about 20 daily units of insulin to about 40 almost overnight. That was my second child Lauren, being loud and making her presence felt from the moment of conception. I was very well researched by that second pregnancy, at 41 years of age. Aside from rapidly increasing insulin requirements, up to about 120 units prior to delivery, it was a totally uneventful pregnancy. My second child was born at 40 weeks by cesarean (related not to diabetes, but to failure to progress with labor due to her being tied up in the umbilical cord and unable to drop). She weighed 7lbs 6 oz and was very healthy, and very loud (she still is to this day). About 15 minutes after delivery, I asked the nurses to give me glucose now! I felt myself going low. They said they needed to get orders from the doctor first. I yelled at them that I would lose consciousness if they didn't act immediately.

Fortunately, they then responded. I was on a glucose drip for several days before my blood sugar stabilized (no wonder, going from about 120 units a day to about 20 units a day with the removal of the placenta).

Low-Carb

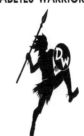

"Thriving, not just surviving."

By the time my third pregnancy had rolled around, I had made a drastic life change. At age 30 I was over 200lb (never lost the baby weight from #2), blood sugars were not well-controlled, and I was taking 15 prescription medications ranging from blood pressure meds and cholesterol meds to antidepressants, sleeping pills and diuretics from the swelling the ACE inhibitor (bp med which was supposed to protect my kidneys) caused.

I discovered the website of a man named Steve Cooksey, the Diabetes Warrior, who had reversed his type 2 diabetes and lost 75lb on a low-carb, paleo-style meal plan. He said this way of eating applied to type 1's as well! Obviously, I could not reverse my type 1 diabetes like he had reversed his type 2, but I could control it much better. Type 1's will ALWAYS require insulin, low carb is not a cure, but we can have dramatically better results when we reduce carbohydrates. If we lower our carbohydrates, we lower our insulin, thereby lowering the risk of highs and lows.

Steve spent numerous hours with me instant messaging and on the phone walking me through the details. I had so many questions and I didn't want to give up my carbs! I had spent my childhood not being allowed to eat candy, cakes, and cookies and I had now been told I could eat whatever I wanted and bolus for it. We see where that got me!

In the first month and a half I only lost 5lb. and I was very discouraged, but Steve encouraged me to stick with it.

After 10 months, I had lost 55lb. and had come off all the meds except the insulin which I cut in half. My blood pressure normalized. My cholesterol normalized. Every health marker improved.

One month after I hit my low weight, I found out I was pregnant again! I vowed to do things differently this time.

A person with diabetes is for all intents and purposes, carbohydrate intolerant. Our bodies do not metabolize carbohydrates properly, even with rapid acting insulin.

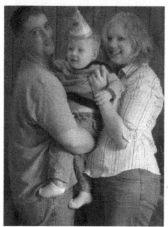

On Aidan's (my second child) 2nd birthday

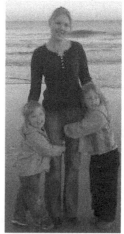

10 months of low carb and 55lb down

So why are we encouraged to eat them? Our bodies make plenty of glucose, so we aren't lacking for fuel. All necessary nutrients can be obtained from sources without sugar or starch.

There is no such thing as a grain deficiency, and carbohydrates are not an essential nutrient. There are essential amino acids (protein), and there are essential fatty acids (fat). If we don't eat these things we'll die, but there is no such thing as an essential carbohydrate. Would you encourage someone who is lactose intolerant to drink milk, or a person who is gluten intolerant to eat wheat? Of course not!

There are reasons your doctor may be against a low-carb diet. There are many myths in the medical community like the idea that saturated fats cause heart disease or that high protein will damage the kidneys. Both of these ideas have been proven untrue in multiple studies. Many medical professionals don't understand nutritional ketosis, and equate it with ketoacidosis. Thankfully, more and more medical professionals are coming around and seeing the benefits of a low carbohydrate diet, but it is a slow shift.

Dr. Bernstein

Steve also introduced me to a book, *Dr. Bernstein's Diabetes Solution.* Dr. Richard Bernstein is a type 1 diabetic of 75 years who was the first to use home blood glucose monitoring and the basal/bolus method of insulin dosing. He discovered that by eating a low-carb, high-protein diet with precise insulin dosing techniques, he was able to essentially have normal blood sugars around the clock! I know this sounds ridiculous for a type 1. I felt the same way. I can remember laughing at type 2's who thought a 150mg/dL (8.3mmol/L) blood sugar was high. "They have no idea!" I thought. Let me tell you, I was proven wrong! I now consider 120 mg/dL (6.7 mmol/L) high.

I continued eating low carb through my pregnancy, breast-feeding and beyond, and I saw a lot of improvement, but I couldn't quite get my blood sugars where I wanted them. I got my a1c's down into the 5's during pregnancy, but they had climbed back up into the 7's and even one 8 afterward, despite eating almost no carbohydrates. I thought I was following Dr. Bernstein, but I actually wasn't. There was so much I was missing.

NATIONAL BESTSELLER

Dr. Bernstein's
DIABETES
SOLUTION

THE COMPLETE GUIDE
TO ACHIEVING NORMAL
BLOOD SUGARS

4ᵀᴴ EDITION,
NEWLY REVISED
& UPDATED

Richard K. Bernstein, MD

So, what do you eat?

I avoid grains, sugar, starch, and sweet fruits. My diet mainly consists of meat, eggs, some dairy (but no milk except Fairlife milk which is low carb, or unsweetened almond milk), non-starchy vegetables, nuts, seeds, and the occasional low-carb baked treat.

I was low carb for my entire pregnancy, and a little over 2 years prior, eating approximately 30g carbs per day. My doctors were ok with me eating low carb, as my A1C was so low. My endocrinologist and OB both commented that it is normal and poses no risks to baby, and that my A1C was probably better than theirs. Their only comment was that low carb during pregnancy has never technically been studied.

-Leah Wornath

Blood Sugar Friendly Foods ☑

PROTEIN	VEGETABLES	
Beef	Asparagus	Eggplant
Chicken	Artichoke	Green Beans
Deli Meat (no sugar)	Avocado	Hearts of Palm
Eggs	Broccoli	Jicama
Egg white Protein	Brussels Sprouts	Kale
Fish	Cabbage	Lettuce (any)
Hemp Protein	Cauliflour (rice)	Okra
Nuts (limit)	Celery	Peppers
Pork	Coconut Aminos	Radish
Seafood	Collard Greens	Spinach
Seeds	Cucumber	Summer Squash
Whey Protein	Daikon Radish	Water Chestnuts
		Zucchini

DAIRY
Almond Milk (unsweetened)
Aldi Keto Ice Cream
Califia Farms Betterhalf
Carb Master Milk
Carb Master Yogurt
Cashew Milk (unsweetened)
Cream Cheese (limit if trying to lose weight).
Coconut milk (read label)
Endulge Keto Ice Cream
Fairlife Milk
Flax Milk (unsweetened)
Heavy Whipping Cream (limit if trying to lose weight)
Half n Half (limit)

Hemp Milk (unsweetened)
Kite Hill almond milk yogurt (plain)
Kite Hill Cream Cheese
Nutpods Creamer
Plain whole fat yogurt (test))
Two-good Yogurt (test)
Plain Coconut Milk Yogurt
Plain YQ Yogurt (test)
Rebel Ice Cream
Real Good No Sugar Added

FATS
Avocado Oil
Butter
Coconut Oil
Ghee
Olive Oil

You can find other blood sugar friendly products and recipes here: http://www.pinterest.com/typeonegrit

Everyone is different. Test all foods to your meter. If the food spikes you more than 20mg/dL (with a bolus) you may need more insulin. If you spike even with increased insulin, you likely need to avoid that food. Yogurt for instance, spikes some people and not others, even with minimal carbohydrates.

I wanted to keep my blood sugars even lower and more stable during the pregnancy, so I committed to repeating the same meals and snacks repeatedly. Variety is not your friend during pregnancy. I had a pretty good first trimester, but I had some major food aversions, and it was very difficult to eat meats and veggies (which usually are 80% of my diet). So, I made some Keto breads/muffins and bought some keto cereals which allowed me to get some substance and feel less nauseous.

Blood Sugar Friendly Foods 2

Homemade dressings
Homemade Mayo
Primal Kitchen dressings
Primal Kitchen Mayo
Oil & Vinegar dressing
Walden Farms dressings
DRINKS
Bai Bubbles
Blue Sky Stevia Sodas
Coffee
Crystal Light
Diet Sodas
Mio Drops
Sparkling Water
Stur Water Flavoring
Tea

PRE-MADE PRODUCTS
All Better Keto Cookies (no fruit)
Awesome Bunz
Bake Believe Chocolate Chips
Better Than Noodles/Rice
Cali'flour Pizza Crusts
Cereal School cereals and snacks
Crepini Egg Thins
Evolved Keto Cups
Flackers
G. Hughes BBQ Sauce
Guy's BBQ Sauce
Heinz "no sugar added" ketchup
High Key Cereals and Cookies
Keto and Co. Pancake/Waffle Mix
Know Foods Cookies
Lankanto Maple Flavored Syrup

Water
Zevia Sodas
SWEETENERS
Allulose
Bochasweet
Liquid Monk Fruit Extract
Lankanto and Whole Earth
Monk Fruit Sweetener
Stevia drops
Truvia (not baking blend)
Sweet Additions
stevia/erythritol blend
Swerve (erythritol)
Pyure (stevia and erythritol)
Splenda Zero (liquid)
Liquid Sucralose
Stevia Extract (read label)
Lily's Chocolate
Max Mallow
Miracle Flour (lupin)
Moon Cheese
Nuco Coconut Wraps
Palmini Noodles
Rao's Pasta Sauce
Real Good Products (not cauli crust pizza)
Plantpower Sandwich Thins
Quest Chips/Cookies/Pizza
Shrewd Food Protein Crisps
Smart Buns
Superfat Keto Cookies
Tasty Pastry
Think Keto Protein Bars
Walden Farms Products

By the second trimester, I was able to eat more substance, and I had a very repetitive diet. Breakfast was 2.5 hours after I woke up to avoid the morning insulin resistance. I would have 3 pasture raised eggs slightly runny. Lunch was grass-fed taco meat or pork sausage with some cheese. Dinner was always a large salad with EVOO (extra-virgin olive oil), chicken or chicken sausage, or more grass-fed beef. Occasionally I did fish or we would eat out and I would order something very low carb. For snacks I had nuts, seeds, cheese, low carb yogurt, Lily's chocolate or occasionally keto bread or keto cereal. This was my diet 95% of my second and third trimesters, and keeping the food repetitive really helped me focus on the dosing adjustments for the hormonal insulin resistance that occurs over the course of the pregnancy.

-Olivia

What if I'm vegetarian or vegan?

If you eat eggs and dairy as a vegetarian, it's pretty easy, but it's more difficult as a vegan. It can be done, however. The focus needs to be on getting adequate protein and fat.

Norma Plum is a type 1 who eats low-carb vegan. She had a healthy pregnancy, and her baby had no complications.

> I'm petite and don't eat much. I'm always back to my pre-pregnancy weight the day after I give birth. I know, lucky me. I ate lots of tofu scrambles with all kinds of greens: kale, chard, spinach. Huge salads with stir fried veggies - mushrooms, onions, broccoli, and avocados. I snack on nuts and seeds. I ate lots of pickles with hummus, and sauerkraut. Some vegan meat substitutes occasionally (like tofurky Italian sausage with sauerkraut).

Norma struggled with her dietitian pushing back.

> The dietitian just pushed carbs all the time. She wanted me to eat rice, tortillas, and bread. She didn't like that I ate so much avocado. My weight was very well controlled. I don't think I put on more than 2 lbs. a month.

> When I explained to her that healthy fats are good for the baby's brain, she dismissed me.

There is some question about soy, as it can be goitrogenic (affects the function of the thyroid) and contains phytoestrogens. Like anything else, this is a personal decision.

TypeOneGrit

In 2014 I met some amazing people in the Facebook Dr. Bernstein group; R.D. Dikeman, who is a theoretical physicist and father of a type one son, Debbie Theriault, who is a fitness guru and nutrition coach who was diagnosed t1 as an adult, and Derek Raulerson, who is a lifelong type 1 and a father to a type 1 son as well. We were like minded and decided to start a group for type 1 diabetics and parents of type 1 diabetics who follow Dr. Bernstein, and thus TypeOneGrit was born.

The group has grown to over 3000 members worldwide, we have more than 25,000 followers on Facebook to date, and our group has been featured in two studies: one by Duke University and one by Harvard. The studies showed amazing results. Our group's average a1c was 5.5%. No diabetes medication or technology can come close to this. Another thing the study found; the higher the carbs, the higher the a1c.

So, I finally read Dr. Bernstein's book cover to cover. It is a long read. I compare it to the Bible. I find it more useful to use it as a resource guide than a straight read. I use the search feature in the eBook to find whatever I need to look up. It turns out that even though I was eating low-carb, I was not following Dr. Bernstein's protocols.

Bolusing Protein?

A big aspect I was missing was bolusing for protein. When we are educated in diabetes management, nobody ever mentions that we need insulin for protein, but it's true.

The thing is, when we are eating a lot of carbohydrate, and taking a lot of insulin to cover that carbohydrate, the protein rise gets lost in the mix. When we remove the carbs, it becomes apparent.

There is a big myth in the low-carb world that protein is turning to sugar and should therefore be severely limited. Nothing could be further from the truth! Protein should be the focus here. To clarify, protein *is* converted to glucose via gluconeogenesis, but this is a slow, continual process. The spike you see post-meal is not from the protein becoming glucose; rather, it is due to a glucagon response.

In a normal, healthy, non-diabetic person, when protein is ingested it is broken down into amino acids and the body responds with a glucagon and insulin response.

Remember Glucagon? That scary needle that comes in a red or orange case, that is to be used if you pass out from low blood sugar? Same thing. Glucagon signals your liver to release glucose from the glycogen stores, and the insulin balances it out. The problem is when your insulin doesn't work, or you don't make any! For this reason, insulin needs to be injected when eating protein, to keep that Glucagon in check.

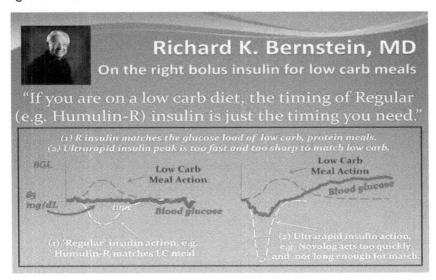

Dr. Bernstein recommends using R (regular) insulin (which can be purchased over the counter at Walmart for $25) to cover protein as it has a slower onset and longer duration than the rapid-acting insulins. Dr. B. gives us a starting point of ½ unit or R insulin per oz of protein food. This is *just* a starting point as everyone is different. Most people need to pre-bolus R insulin by around 45 minutes before the meal. I personally have to give R an hour to an hour and a half *after* my meal. You'll need to experiment to see how fast R becomes active in your system and how long it takes for you to see a protein spike. This is all explained in Dr. Bernstein's book, *Dr. Bernstein's Diabetes Solution.*

Rapid-acting insulin is used for corrections, or when you can't wait the 45 minutes it takes for the R to kick in before eating (say, at a restaurant). Most doctors don't use R insulin anymore and are honestly unable to advise on dosing it for the most part, so usually don't recommend using it. The R action profile can be mimicked with strategic dosing, such as injecting Humalog around 2 hours post-meal when I start to see an upward trend on my Dexcom). A starting place for covering protein with rapid acting insulin is half the insulin of your insulin to carb ratio, so if you take say, 1 unit for 10g of carbohydrate, you might take ½ unit per 10g of protein. Again, this is a *very* individual thing that takes a lot of trial and error to master. Some use a square-wave bolus on their pump to mimic R.

Another thing I was missing was splitting my basal insulin. Most of us on MDI (multiple daily injections) are instructed to take one big dose of Lantus/ Levemir/Tresiba to cover the next 24 hours, but in Dr. Bernstein's opinion, "there is no 24-hour insulin". He even splits Tresiba. Some people do well on a single dose though. This is very individual so work with your physician on this.

Dr. B. also recommends an ideal blood sugar of 83mg/dL (outside pregnancy). I wasn't correcting until 140 mg/dL (7.7 mmol/L) or so prior to this, so of course my a1c wasn't where I wanted it. I now have my high alert on my Dexcom set to 120mg/dL (6.7mmol/L) which is as low as you can set it, and I'll even do an IM shot for a 120.

One of the biggest tenets of Dr. Bernstein's plan is the *Law of Small Numbers.* "Big inputs make big mistakes; small inputs make small mistakes." Large amounts of carbohydrate are unpredictable. Like I said before, nutrition labels are allowed to be up to 20% off and even if they were absolutely accurate, how they are absorbed varies day to day, minute to minute. Insulin absorption also varies, so it's very rare that you're going to match them up perfectly. You're likely going to go too high or too low with large amounts of carbs. With small amounts of carbs, we're taking small amounts of insulin, so we're less likely to go high or low. If we are off on our carbs or insulin slightly, we might go a tiny bit high or low, which is easily corrected.

There are many other aspects to this protocol, so please read the book for yourself! It is available on Amazon, you can buy it used on Bookfinder.com, you can check out from your library, or you can buy the eBook. If you have trouble getting Dr. Bernstein's book, feel free to contact me, and I will make sure you can get a copy.

Won't high protein damage my kidneys?

High protein doesn't damage healthy kidneys. High blood sugars damage healthy kidneys. This myth has been perpetuated for decades based on a faulty study. Dr.

Bernstein tells the story: "The restriction of protein intake is old, old time. It was born of a study by Barry Brenner at Harvard back in the 80s. He did a survey of the diabetologists in Boston: "Where do you like to keep your diabetics? What blood sugar?" And they said 250. So, he said, I'm going to clamp my rats at 250 and put half on ordinary rat chow and half on a high-protein diet. All the rats died of rat kidney disease, diabetic kidney disease, but those on the high-protein diet died twice as fast. He got funding that enabled him to travel around the country boasting of this discovery.

He went to the ADA people in New York and said: "Do you like to keep your patient's blood sugars at 250?" They all raised their hands. But I stood up and challenged it. I said, "Diabetics are entitled to normal blood sugars." And I got booed.

That was the end of it as far as the general medical population knows. But five years later, I was collaborating on a study with the top guy in hyper-tension in the New York area. Very famous fellow, he pushed development of the ACE inhibitors. And his research fellow and I were working on a study that involved kidney function. He presented the results at a kidney conference in Washington DC. And on the agenda for the same day was Barry Brenner. Brenner repeated his study with rats and this time clamped their blood sugars at 90. No rats died of kidney disease – they all lived healthy rat lives. That got published in the abstracts of this meeting. Long gone, it never hit the general population. Harvard did not pay for press releases or for a tour around the country. But he proved that he was wrong."

Numerous studies in the last few years have shown NO correlation between high protein diets and kidney disease, yet the myth continues. Dr. Bernstein himself was able to reverse his Stage 3 Chronic Kidney Disease by following his low carb high protein diet. If you are to the point of almost needing dialysis, then yes, protein should be restricted.

Getting the Green Light to Conceive

What should your a1c be? It depends on who you ask. Most will say less than 7% for trying to conceive and less than 6.5% for pregnancy. According to the American Diabetes Association, it should be between 6.0 and 6.5% for pregnancy. If it is possible to lower a1c below 6%, this is recommended. ACOG (American College of Obstetrics and Gynecology) recommends less than 6%. Dr. Bernstein's targets are lower. According to Dr. B., non-diabetic pregnant women run in the 60's fasting, so target a1c should be in the 4's.

Dr. Lois Jovanovich, who was a world-renowned endocrinologist who specialized in pregnancy and diabetes would not allow her patients to get pregnant until their a1c matched their non-diabetic partner's a1c. A good method if you ask me.

It's recommended to get the "green light" from your endocrinologist before you try to conceive. I personally was never actually trying. I had been "practicing" tracking my ovulation, temping etc. and in actuality I really was trying, but I didn't think I could get pregnant. Therefore, my a1c was not at all optimal for pregnancy. The same went for my second pregnancy. I was tracking, but not actively trying. Number 3 was a total surprise. Even though I was eating low carb with him, my A1c was something like 7.3%. I was low carb, but not yet following Dr. Bernstein.

Table 6.5 Glucose Targets in Pregnancy

	A1C (%)	Premeal Glucose (mg/dl)	Postmeal Glucose (mg/dl)	Nocturnal (mg/dl)
ADA[19]	<6.0	60–99	100–129 peak postprandial	—
ACOG[75]	<6.0	Fasting: 95 Premeal: 100	1 h: <140 2 h: <120	60
NICE[76]	Not recommended in second and third trimester	63–106	1 h: <140	—
Canada[22]	—	68–94	1 h: 99–139 2 h: 90–119	>65
Australia[77]	"within the normal range"	72–99	1 h: <144 2 h: <126	
IDF[78]	<6.0	60–120		

Photo from http://www.diabetesincontrol.com/adajdrf-type-1-diabetes-sourcebok-excerpt-13-setting-treatment-targets-part-2-of-2/

Again, I thought I was following Bernstein because I was low carb, but I wasn't. With each pregnancy I was able to get my a1c down quickly and was in the 5's for the majority of my pregnancies.

The Rules for the 5 or Less Club

So how do you get your blood sugars under control so you can get that green light to conceive?

Over the years I put together a list of tips and tricks that helped me to get my a1c into the 5's or below. I've had many people advise me based on their experience, the major ones being Steve Cooksey, RD Dikeman, Debbie Theriault, Derek Raulerson, Doris Dickson, and Lisa La Nasa (my current employer at diaVerge!) These tips were super helpful, and I hope they will help you as well.

First and foremost, read **"Dr. Bernstein's Diabetes Solution".** There are many factors, but the main ones include:

- No more than 30g of carbs per day. I get my carbs from non-starchy vegetables and nuts/seeds. Keep them right around this number though. Lower is not always better. When I am near zero carb, I become insulin resistant.

- I eat no carbs if bg is over 110mg/dL (6.1 mmol/L). Eat protein and fat.

- Target to 83mg/dL (4.6 mmol/L). I recommend targeting 70mg/dL(3.8mmol/L) for pregnancy.

- When blood sugar is low, correct only to target. To do this you need to find out exactly how much 1g of carbohydrate raises you. Eat a set number of carbs, say 10g and see how high it raises you. Do this fasting, with a stable blood sugar and no insulin on board. This will show you how much 1g raises you and you can adjust your insulin to carb ratio based on this. 1g raises me around 5mg/dL so if I were say, 60 (3.3) and wanted to be 80 (4.4) I would take 4g of carb in the form of glucose tabs, liquid glucose, American Smarties (Rockets in Canada, Fizzers in AU) Sweet Tarts, Bottlecaps or Spree only. Don't treat low blood sugar with food.

- When eating low carb, you get your needed glucose from protein via hepatic gluconeogenesis. While this provides needed glucose, the spike you see after meals is surprisingly not from GNG. When we eat protein, and it is broken down into amino acids, this causes an insulin/glucagon response. In a normal, healthy, non-diabetic, the insulin and glucagon balance out, but in a diabetic, the glucagon works, but the insulin doesn't (or there isn't any!) This causes a spike typically 2-3 hours post meal and needs to be covered with insulin. Many find using R insulin works beautifully, while others prefer to use rapid acting after the fact. Either is fine.

- Find out exactly how much 1 unit drops you so you can correct to target. This is your correction factor or sensitivity. I do this on an empty stomach with no active rapid insulin on board. I do this when blood sugar is on the higher end, say, 140mg/dL (7.7mmol/L) but not excessively high as this causes more insulin resistance. Test at 30 minutes, 1hr. and 2hr. and see how much the 1 unit dropped you. If you are insulin sensitive, use ½ a unit.

- I wear a Dexcom and correct often with micro-boluses. I correct at 95mg/ dL (5.2) on the pump and at 100mg/dL (5.5) on MDI (I use 3/10 cc syringes with half unit markings.) You can also dilute insulin to micro-bolus. Diluent is free from the manufacturer and does not require a prescription, though it does need to be sent to a pharmacy, clinic, or hospital.

- Download Dexcom Clarity every 3 days at least to look for patterns. If you don't use a cgm, download your meter or pump.

- Do 24-hour basal testing to make sure your basal rates (or long-acting insulin) is correct. The idea is to fast for 24 hours and watch what your blood sugar does. You can do this in 4-hour increments if you can't tolerate longer. Test every hour. If you go up by more than 15-30mg/dL (0.8 mmol/L), your basal is too low, if you go down, it is too high.

- If doing MDI (multiple daily injections), I split mylong-acting as it does NOT last 24 hours. Lantus, I do twice a day, morning, and evening. Levemir needs to be split 3 ways for most people. The smaller the dose, the less time it will last.

- http://www.diabetes-book.com/opinion-no-24-hour-basal-insulin/ Dr. Bernstein is even splitting Tresiba, though some people do fine with one dose of Tresiba.

- Insulin sensitizing supplements can be helpful. I've had good results with R-Alpha Lipoic Acid, Biotin, Chromium and Zinc. Dr. B also recommends Evening Primrose Oil. Metformin can be very helpful as well. It's not just for t2's. Metformin is also helpful in PCOS and has actually shown to help prevent miscarriage in women with PCOS. It can also help with milk supply. Discuss Metformin with your doctor.

- To bring down highs quickly I inject IM (intramuscularly). I use the deltoid muscle (upper arm, near the shoulder cap) or the vastus lateralis (upper outer thigh). You can read more about this here: http://diatribe.org/ issues/39/thinking-like-a-pancreas Dr. B. also has a video on this on his YouTube channel, Diabetes University.

- To prevent false hypos (the symptoms of hypoglycemia despite normal bg), slowly lower your target. For example, if you have been running 180mg/dL (10mmol/L), lower target to 160mg/dL (8.8 mmol/L) for a week, then 140mg/dL (7.7 mmol/L) for a week and so on. If proliferative retinopathy is present, Dr. Bernstein recommends checking IGF-1 levels and if they are elevated, bring your target down slowly. This test should be repeated every couple months.

- Ketones don't worry me if I am healthy and bg is normal. I don't waste my time checking them except in the case of very high bg (over 250mg/dL) or dehydrating illness. Nutritional ketosis is a very healthy state and doesn't need to be feared. If you are taking an SGLT-2 Inhibitor, this is a different story. That said, Dr. Bernstein's plan is not a ketogenic diet.

- Insulin needs go up post ovulation, then again right before my cycle starts. I need to increase my basal insulin during these times. You'll see the same thing in early pregnancy as progesterone levels rise. Metformin is also helpful during this period of time.

- I test frequently if not on cgm and correct aggressively.

- I pre-bolus my meals at least 15 min if possible, with rapid acting insulin. R insulin typically needs a 45-minute pre-bolus, though this is highly individual. I watch the Dexcom for my blood sugar to drop, then I eat. This time can be as much as 45 minutes to an hour for rapid-acting insulin during pregnancy.

- I eat my protein and fat first, then my veggies. The protein and fat slow down the carbs and give the insulin time to kick in.

- Weight training raises me, cardio lowers, so I do weights, then cardio to bring it back down. This works best with a tiny bit of IOB (insulin on board). If you are only doing cardio, I recommend exercising fasted with no insulin on board to avoid lows. Carry liquid glucose to use as needed throughout your workout.

Is Your Basal Too High?

- If you drop overnight, basal is likely too high.

- If you drop when you miss a meal, basal is likely too high.

- If you find a food with carbohydrates "doesn't spike", your basal is likely too high.

- If you don't need to cover protein, your basal is likely too high.

- If you see negative IOB (insulin on board) on your loop, basal is too high.

Basal Testing

As stated previously, basal insulin is your *background* insulin that if given at the correct dose, should keep blood sugars relatively flat in the fasting state. Basal covers the fasting state. Let me repeat that, *basal covers the fasting state.* It has **nothing** to do with food. If your basal is set correctly, your blood sugar should not drop if you were to skip a meal. On the other hand, if you can eat something with carbohydrate or protein and your blood sugar doesn't rise, you likely are taking too much basal.

So how do we test if the basal dose is accurate? By fasting. Optimally the fast lasts for 24 hours. If you can't tolerate 24, you can do 12. If you can't tolerate that, you can do it over multiple days. Skip breakfast the first day (you've also been fasting all night so can measure that as well). The next day, eat breakfast as normal, but skip lunch and have a late dinner if you can. The next day, have a late lunch and skip dinner.

Start the test on an empty stomach at least 4 hours after a meal and/or bolus.

Do this on a day you are not working out. We don't want exercise changing basal needs.

Test every hour for at least a 4-hour period.

For overnight basal testing, if you have a cgm you can just look at your overnight readings the next morning. If you don't use a cgm, you'll need to test every 2 hours during the night. If blood sugar rises more than say 15-30mg/dL (or 1 to 2 mmol/L for easier math), your basal needs to be increased. If it drops, basal needs to be decreased.

If blood sugar drops below 70mg/dL (or 60mg/dL during pregnancy) stop the test and treat the hypoglycemia. If your blood sugar rises above 200mg/dL/11.1mmol/L (or whatever number, you aren't comfortable rising above) stop the test and treat the high blood sugar.

If you are pregnant, we don't want to be fasting for prolonged periods, so I would recommend splitting the test up and skipping a single meal. Another way to get an idea if basal is set correctly is by eating fixed meals that you know the exact dose for the meal and observing if corrections are needed throughout the day. If you're constantly making corrections for highs, basal is likely too low. If you're constantly treating lows, basal is likely too high. If your blood sugar is high or low within a couple hours of a meal, it's likely bolus related.

Treating Hypoglycemia

A major factor in normalizing my blood sugars came down to how I treated hypoglycemia. In diabetes education, we are taught the "Rule of 15". The rule is simple. If blood glucose drops below 70mg/dL/3.8mmol/L (hypoglycemia) treat with 15g of fast-acting carbohydrate. You're given a list of things that are considered such, like juice, regular soda, hard candy, or other sugary items. You wait 15 minutes and if the blood sugar is still below 70 mg/dL, you give another 15g. This rule is set up to get you out of the danger zone and to get you far from it.

Dr. Bernstein recommends treating hypos with glucose only. Most of us were taught we could use anything sweet, but this leads to unpredictable results as well as "eating the whole kitchen" which will result in high blood sugars.

You can use glucose tabs, liquid glucose, glucose gel, glucose gummies, Smarties (American version), Sweet Tarts, Spree, or Bottle Caps. These candies are all dextrose based.

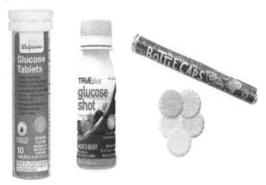

He also recommends treating to target rather than the blanket, "Rule of 15". Say I'm 60 mg/dL (3.3 mmol/L) and I want to be 85 (4.7 mmol/L). I know that 1g of glucose will raise me 5 mg/dL. I need to go up 25 mg/dL so I would need 5g of glucose to raise me to 85mg/dL. If I were to eat 15g, it would spike me to 135mg/dL which is too high.

My personal favorite hypo treatment is liquid glucose. It is the fastest method I have found by far. I use Elovate dextrose packets. CVS also sells glucose packets, or you can buy a big bag of dextrose online or from a health food store. The Elovate packets come in 15 g of dextrose which as I've said before, is typically too much. I split it up into 3 bottles (I buy little glass bottles, add water and shake. This works much faster than glucose tabs or candy.)

Sometimes you may not have glucose or dextrose candies available. Maybe you had a bad day of lows and you ran through your supply. In this situation, treat with whatever you have available, whether it be juice, soda, lifesavers, skittles, maple syrup, honey, or even cake icing. While these treatments are not optimal, they will work in a pinch. One of the reasons we recommend only treating with glucose is the fact that glucose is a simple sugar.

Things like honey, soda, skittles, and maple syrup have fructose in addition to the glucose that must be shunted to the liver first, so they will take longer. Avoid things like chocolate as it has added fat which will delay the absorption of the glucose as well.

You can estimate glucose needs by weight. There is a chart in Dr. Bernstein's book that estimates how much 1g of glucose will raise blood sugar. This number won't always work. If you have a large amount of insulin on board that shouldn't be there, such as making a big dosing error (much more unlikely on low carb, but late in pregnancy, you will likely be taking large doses) or if basal is set too high. If you treat a low and blood sugar rises, but then drops back down, it's likely too much basal.

For those of us following Dr. Bernstein, we know that 15g is almost always too much (unless we've made a large dosing error, which is unlikely) and will raise blood sugar to unacceptable levels. Low-carbers tend to be more sensitive to carbohydrate also, so they tend to need less to treat. What number do you use then? Your glucose sensitivity number! We want to find out exactly how much 1g of glucose will raise your blood sugar so we can treat precisely to target (83mg/dL or 4.6mmol/dL outside of pregnancy). The best way to do this is to find out exactly how much 1g. raises you.

Four hours after your last bolus:

- Take a designated amount of glucose. (I used 10g for easy math, but you can use whatever you're comfortable with)

- Do this on an empty stomach during the day (b.g.'s fluctuate in the morning), on an empty stomach, with no active insulin on board (rapid acting).

- We want to do this when blood sugar is at a lower number, but not low, say around 70-80mg/dL, or 3.8mmo/L-4.4mmol/L).

- Test at 30 minutes, 1 hr. and 2 hr. and see how high you go. From this you can determine how much 1g of glucose raises your blood sugar. You'll see the majority of the action by 1 hour, but I say 2 hours to be thorough, plus it will act as a "mini" basal test. For instance, some people might rise from the glucose, but by the 2-hour mark, their blood sugar has dropped back down. This tells me their basal is likely too high.

I tested the 10g and after 1 hour my blood glucose had risen 50mg/dL or 2.7mmol/L, so I knew that 1g raises me 5mg/dL or 0.27mmol/L. By doing this, you can treat to target and not over treat your lows and get on the roller coaster. It is not *necessary* to use 10g. I just used it for easy math. Use whatever amount you're comfortable with.

If you are like I was, and are used to treating lows with cereal, or whatever you can get your hands on, this can be a big adjustment. I put Smarties out everywhere; beside my bed, in the bathroom, in the kitchen, in my car, any place I could think of, so I would remember to use glucose instead of food. I had to train myself to think of glucose as medicine, and not a fun treat that I get to have when I'm low (a good way to overtreat).

Testing Insulin Sensitivity

In addition to treating hypoglycemia to target, we want to treat *hyperglycemia* (high blood sugar) to target as well. Most type 1's using MDI, or an insulin pump use a correction factor, or insulin sensitivity number to make corrections. For instance, 1 unit lowers blood glucose by 50mg/dL or 2.7mmol/L. This is typically an arbitrary number assigned by your doctor and is adjusted as needed. We can treat highs *precisely* by knowing exactly how much 1 unit lowers blood glucose. Now for this to be accurate, we need basal to be accurate, so I recommend doing basal testing first.

- Again, we do this on an empty stomach with no active rapid acting on board (at least 4 hours after your last bolus).

- This time we do the test at a *higher* number, but not super high, say around 150mg/dL or 8 mmol/L for easy math.

- We take 1 unit and measure how much the insulin drops the blood sugar over 4 hours. The majority of the glucose lowering will happen in the first two hours, but for a full picture, we want to test for 4 hours.

- Once we have this number, we can make a correction to target. 1 unit lowers my blood sugar by 85mg/dL, so if I were 150mg/dL (8.3mmol/dL) and want to be 83mg/dL (4.6mmol/L) I would subtract 83 from 150 and divide by 85.

$$150 - 83 = 67 \qquad \text{then:} \qquad \frac{67}{83} = 0.78$$

Now on an insulin pump, I can give precisely 0.78 units but, on a syringe, (with half unit markings) I can only dose in ½ unit increments, so would give 0.5 units. You can mark your syringe in between these lines to get a quarter unit. If you are very sensitive and know that 1 unit will drop you too much, you can use ½ unit or whatever amount you're comfortable with.

Correcting at a lower number

Many diabetics who aren't following Dr. Bernstein will not make a correction until they hit say, 200mg/dL or 11.1 mmol/L or maybe 150mg/dL 8.3mmol/L. During my last pregnancy, though I was eating low carb, I wasn't making corrections until I got to 140mg/dL, even though for pregnancy the post meal target is 120mg/dL or 6.6 mmol/L or less. I recommend setting your high alert on your cgm to 120 so you can make a correction before you actually become high. Once blood sugar rises above 180mg/dL or so, blood sugars are much harder to bring down, but high glucose or glucose toxicity, causes insulin resistance. If you have ketones, it's even more difficult.

Chapter 3: PCOS

I'm hoping to become pregnant within the next year. I am 30, have no children, and have never been pregnant. I see my endo in a couple weeks and was considering asking for a maternal fetal medicine consult. I also have PCOS and am kind of worried I'll have difficulty conceiving.

I'm pretty clueless on what I should be doing right now. I'm hoping my endo will let me know if I need to be taking any supplements or what else I can do. I've been off birth control pills for a month. The good news is my A1c has been between 4.8-5.0 for the past year and a half. So at least that part of my body is ready.

What is PCOS?

PCOS or polycystic ovarian syndrome is a disorder in which a woman's adrenal glands produce more male hormones (testosterone) than they should. This can cause a myriad of problems. These problems include:

- Irregular Periods Long, heavy periods
- Hirsutism (having a lot of hair where you shouldn't such as your face.
- Insulin Resistance (high testosterone in women can be caused by high insulin levels).
- Weight Gain
- Acne
- Acanthosis Nigricans (darkening of the skin on the back of the neck, the axilla (underarms), joints of the fingers and the genital area).
- Male-Pattern Baldness
- Thinning Hair
- Fatigue
- Low Sex-drive
- Infertility

Treatment for PCOS includes Metformin (a drug that makes you more sensitive to insulin, thereby lowering insulin, thereby lowering testosterone), Spironolactone (a potassium sparing diuretic that lowers testosterone and can help with things like the facial hair and acne), and birth control pills. Dr. Bernstein uses Metformin, TNF Alpha inhibitors, Ramipril (an ACE inhibitor) along with some of the supplements he mentions for insulin resistance such as R-fraction Alpha Lipoic Acid, Vitamin E and Evening Primrose Oil.

Some studies have shown that a low-carb diet can increase fertility in women with PCOS. This makes sense for the same reason the Metformin makes sense. If you decrease your carbs, you decrease your insulin and decrease your testosterone. Metformin has also shown to prevent miscarriage when taken in pregnancy for women with PCOS.

I personally have PCOS, which is probably why it took me 3 years before I got pregnant, even though I wasn't on birth control. I actually got pregnant with all 3 of my babies while on a low-carb diet. With my first I was doing the Atkins Diet to lose weight, and with my second, I was doing Atkins to lose the baby weight. By the time number three came along I was doing this lifelong low carb. I've now been eating this way for eleven years! It is absolutely sustainable in the long term!

Chapter 4: The Safety of Low Carb in Pregnancy

The pregnancy was a surprise, but I was thrilled. I had always wanted three children and this time I was going to do it the right way! I continued eating low carb/paleo throughout my pregnancy and had the easiest of my three pregnancies with absolutely no complications. He was my only child to go to a full 40 weeks, and his birth was a vaginal birth after two cesareans, which is almost unheard of in a type 1 diabetic (it's rare in any pregnancy). Steve Cooksey was a huge help throughout my pregnancy.

Doesn't Baby Need Carbs to Grow?

This is the biggest question I encounter. I also hear an uproar from obstetricians and CDE's. Baby needs carbs to grow! What exactly are they basing this on? I think there is some slight confusion of terms. Baby needs *glucose* to grow, not carbohydrate. Say I eat a piece of bread. The piece of bread does not go to the baby. As soon as I start chewing, the enzymes in my saliva start breaking the bread down into glucose, while it's still in my mouth!

You can actually test this out. Buy some Diastix on Amazon. These used to be used to test a diabetic's urine for glucose before we had meters. Put the bread in your mouth and start chewing. Get it good and mixed up with your saliva, then place the strip in your mouth. Within seconds it will have turned black because it is already converting to glucose! So, my body absorbs the glucose into my bloodstream, and the baby gets a constant flow of glucose through the placenta from my bloodstream.

Say I don't eat any carbs except vegetables (this is what I do). My body converts the protein and even the fat if necessary, into glucose via hepatic gluconeogenesis.

Here's a question for you. As a type 1 diabetic, what happens if you forget your basal insulin shot or if your pump malfunctions and you don't get insulin? You got it; your blood sugar rapidly increases! Why? Because your body is making glucose all on its own! So, if there is at least a normal amount of sugar in your blood (or even less than normal, but we'll talk about that later) your baby will get the glucose it needs whether you eat carbohydrate or not. Of course, we want plenty of vegetables for nutrients.

What About Ketones?

This is the next topic the doctors jump to. Ketones! As a t1, I'm sure you know about ketones. For those reading who aren't type 1 diabetic, ketones are a byproduct of burned fat. When there is an insulin deficiency, the body can't use glucose (sugar) for fuel, and is in essence, *starving*, so it starts breaking down its own muscle and fat for fuel. The result of this burned fat is ketones. In the absence of insulin, ketones quickly spiral out of control and lower the pH of the blood making it acidic. The person has high blood glucose due to the lack of insulin and the body tries to push the glucose (sugar) out through the urine.

This excessive urination causes dehydration, which exacerbates the situation and makes the ketones higher. DKA (diabetic ketoacidosis) is a very dangerous condition (fatal if untreated). Symptoms include nausea, vomiting, abdominal cramps, lethargy, shortness of breath, and if left untreated, coma and death. DKA typically happens when a basal insulin dose is missed, an insulin pump malfunctions, during illness (when insulin needs increase) and when dehydrated (or both).

The big difference here is insulin. If there is adequate insulin present, ketones are regulated. Insulin keeps them from spinning out of control. If there is no insulin (or not enough) that's where we get into the scary acidic blood, dangerous condition that is an emergency.

What about when there *is* insulin? You've probably heard of a ketogenic diet. Dr. Bernstein's plan is often confused with a ketogenic diet because it is low carb. In a ketogenic diet, the carbs are reduced, and the fat is increased to induce ketosis. The person is making ketones as a result of burning their own fat and ingested fat. Ketosis is a perfectly healthy state if there is adequate insulin on board.

As a type 1 you've probably been taught that ketones are bad. Toxic. They turn your blood into acid. You've probably been instructed to measure them if your blood sugar goes above a certain number, say 250mg/dL or if you are sick and vomiting. This is what first comes to your doctor's mind when he hears the word ketones as well.

Let me preface this by repeating that Dr. Bernstein's plan is NOT a ketogenic diet. It is low-carb, high-protein, and is not high-fat. I personally rarely if ever have ketones. If you are showing ketones, try increasing your protein and

non-starchy vegetables. Ketones are not the goal here, but they aren't scary either. I just wanted to drive home the fact that they aren't dangerous. We evolved on ketones.

The high-carbohydrate diet is the experiment! We know that high blood sugars are teratogenic (harmful to the fetus), so in my opinion, we should be doing whatever is necessary to normalize blood sugars.

One major issue is that healthcare professionals don't know the difference between Nutritional Ketosis and Diabetic Ketoacidosis (DKA). Nutritional ketosis is a natural, healthy state, in which the body is burning fat for fuel instead of carbohydrate, and the byproduct of this burned fat is ketones. People on a ketogenic diet actually check their urine or blood for ketones because that shows they are burning fat for fuel!

So, if you're taking your insulin as needed, blood glucose is normal and you are well-hydrated, ketones are not an issue. A time that ketones *can* present a problem is during illness. If you are vomiting, you can quickly become dehydrated, and because you aren't eating due to the vomiting, you are producing what we call, 'starvation ketones'. Also, during illness, our insulin needs are increased (which will be evidenced by high blood sugars). Hydration and normalization of blood glucose are key here. Try and eat something if you can, and if you can't keep anything down, you may need to go into the emergency room for fluids.

The only caveat here is if you are on SGLT-2 Inhibitors, a class of medication that causes you to pass more glucose through your urine at a lower threshold. The problem with these medications is twofold. One, you are peeing a lot and can become dehydrated. Two, you are lowering your blood sugar by peeing it out, but the issue of too little insulin is present even if your glucose is normal, so you can go into a condition called euglycemic ketoacidosis. SGLT-2 Inhibitors are not approved for pregnancy.

One other thing I want to mention is that the *very* few cases of euglycemic dka (diabetic ketoacidosis with normal blood sugar) that I have seen have almost without fail, been in association with prolonged fasting, something that would *not* be recommended during pregnancy, nor do I recommend for a type 1 diabetic in general. Prolonged fasting causes glycogen (stored glucose) stores in the liver to become depleted, and insulin needs will decrease due to this. Because there is no glycogen, blood sugar levels will be low or normal, but there is not adequate insulin on board (insulin does more than keep blood sugars in check) and we know that with insulin deficiency comes unregulated ketones, which are bad news. When we combine prolonged fasting with dehydrating illness, we are brewing trouble. Other dehydrating situations like nursing a baby combined with prolonged fasting have also led to EDKA.

Different levels of ketones are produced under different circumstances. In my experience as a nurse and CDE, people in DKA have very high ketones, many around 50

mmol/L or more. Some will be lower, at say 10mmol/L. Ketones in the 1-3mmol/L range are the 'optimal' ketone range for people following a ketogenic diet (again, Dr. Bernstein's diet is not a ketogenic diet.)

It is a good idea to have a blood ketone meter on hand in case of pump malfunction or dehydrating illness. Urine ketone strips are not very accurate as the urine may be hours old or concentrated. They also only give a range rather than an exact number, and they measure a different type of ketones than blood meters do. If you are not able to get a blood ketone meter, urine ketone strips are definitely better than nothing.

There have not been many studies on ketosis and pregnancy. The studies we have, generally do not apply to nutritional ketosis. There are rat studies (I'm not a rat, are you?) where the rats are fed a high-fat ketogenic diet with nasty hydrogenated fats. They're not fed healthy fats like avocado oil or olive oil, and definitely not a diet high in protein and lots of vegetables that include nutrients which are imperative for a healthy baby.

Doctors and dietitians frequently warn against low carbohydrate diets in pregnancy, citing a risk of ketosis and that it can potentially harm fetal brain development. There are a few problems with this notion.

First of all, it has never been proven that there is a minimum requirement of carbohydrates during pregnancy; many cultures naturally eat a lower carbohydrate diet and have no trouble having healthy pregnancies and healthy babies. Among a worldwide study of over 200

modern-living hunter gatherer populations, average carbohydrate intake was only 16-22% of calories; this is a far cry from the 45-65% of calories in our dietary guidelines.

Second, only diabetic ketoacidosis and starvation ketosis have been proven harmful to fetal brain development and pregnancy outcomes, not nutritional ketosis. Pregnancy is naturally a state where women more easily go into nutritional ketosis, particularly between meals or an overnight fast (the same type of ketosis that would be induced by a lower carbohydrate diet in someone with well-managed blood sugar who either produces adequate insulin or in a type 1 diabetic taking sufficient insulin).

Nutritional ketosis in a woman who is eating adequate calories, protein, and micronutrients is not equivalent to DKA or starvation ketosis; it is a physiologically normal state in pregnancy.

Finally, ketones provide essential cerebral lipids for fetal brain development and supply approximately 30% of fetal brain energy needs. Babies are born in ketosis and remain in ketosis for at least the first month of life in breastfed infants. Ketones present at low, physiologic levels in pregnancy do not pose a harm to fetal brain development; rather, they appear to be vital to healthy brain development. I explain this thoroughly with all relevant research in chapter 11 of my book, Real Food for Gestational Diabetes.

- Lily Nichols, RDN, CDCES

There are studies on pregnant women who are making ketones due to starvation. I can't imagine starvation would have a positive effect on the baby. There are also studies on diabetic ketoacidosis, which obviously is dangerous. I am not aware of any studies on women following a healthy, nutrient-dense low-carbohydrate diet.

Ketosis is a natural state that is more easily attained during pregnancy. Pregnant women tend to go into ketosis much more quickly than non-pregnant. Women who experience morning-sickness almost definitely have ketones, yet their babies are perfectly healthy. Ketones are naturally present in the placenta and umbilical cord blood of newborns (Muneta, et al., 2018) and infants who are breast-fed are naturally in ketosis (Rooy & Hawdon, 2002).

Nutrition

When I say low carb, I am not referring to a meal plan of bacon and cheese (though these are fine to implement in a healthy diet). This is not the time for "dirty keto" (a ketogenic diet that consists of bun-less bacon cheeseburgers, low-carb protein bars, Diet soda, fat bombs and keto desserts). We want a meal plan with plenty of protein, healthy fats, and lots of vegetables for the nutrients. Dietitians tend to claim that low-carb diets are devoid of nutrients, but if done the right way, this way of eating has *more* nutrients than a standard American diet.

Here are some examples of how nutrients are obtained on a low-carb diet:

- Vitamin A: liver, cod liver oil, broccoli, butter, kale, spinach, collard greens, some cheeses, egg.
- Vitamin B1: pork, sunflower seeds, asparagus, kale, cauliflower, liver, and eggs.

- Vitamin B2: asparagus, cottage cheese, meat, eggs, fish, and green beans.
- Vitamin B3: liver, heart, kidney, chicken, beef, fish (tuna, salmon), eggs, avocados, leafy vegetables, broccoli, asparagus, nuts, mushrooms.
- Vitamin B5: meats, broccoli, avocados. B6: meats and nuts.
- Vitamin B7: egg yolk, liver, some vegetables.
- Vitamin B9 (aka folate or acid folic): liver, sunflower seeds, avocado, broccoli, dark leafy greens, asparagus, nuts, cauliflower.
- Vitamin B12: fish, shellfish, meat, poultry, eggs, and dairy products. C: peppers, liver, kale, broccoli, cauliflower, strawberries
- Vitamin D: produced in the skin after exposure to ultraviolet B light from the sun or artificial sources. Also found in fatty fish, eggs, beef liver, and mushrooms.
- Vitamin E: almonds, avocado, eggs, leafy green vegetables.
- Vitamin K: leafy green vegetables, avocado, Brussels sprouts, parsley.
- Omega 3: salmon, tuna, halibut, oysters, avocado, spinach, kale, walnuts.
- Calcium: almond milk, cheeses, spinach, broccoli, clams, beef.
- Iron: clams, oysters, and organ meats like liver, also spinach.
- Zinc: Seafoods like oysters are also zinc-rich, along with spinach, cashews, and dark chocolate.
- Chromium: Processed meats, green beans, romaine lettuce, broccoli, nuts, and egg yolk.
- Magnesium: dark leafy greens, nuts, seeds, fish, avocados, dark chocolate.
- Potassium: almonds, beef, blackberries, broccoli, Brussels sprouts, clams, salmon, tuna, turkey, avocado, spinach, kale, beef.
- Phosphorus: cheese, nuts, veal, mushrooms, scallops, sardines, salmon, shrimp.
- Sodium: salt, cured meat, some cheeses, pickles.
- Fluorine: pickles, spinach, asparagus, avocados, brussels sprouts, cauliflower, cucumber, green leafy vegetables, nuts (especially almonds), seafood, tinned fish.
- Pantothenic Acid: animal liver and kidney, fish, shellfish, pork, chicken, egg yolk, mushrooms, avocados, broccoli.
- Manganese: seafood, leafy greens, hazelnuts
- Copper: leafy greens, including turnip greens, spinach, Swiss chard, kale,

and mustard greens, walnuts, oysters and other shellfish and organ meats (kidneys, liver).

- Selenium: brazil nuts, seafood, fish, pork, beef, lamb, chicken, turkey, mushroom. (Source Unknown)

Even If you don't eat veggies (which you should because they are delicious) you still get a lot of vitamins and nutrients.

3 oz. (85g) beef: Calcium 1%, Iron 12%, Vitamin D 1%, Vitamin B-6 15%, Vitamin B-12 36%, Magnesium 4%

1 large egg: Vitamin A 5%, Calcium 2%, Iron 3%, Vitamin D 11%, Vitamin B-6 5%, Vitamin B-12 10%, Magnesium 1%

1 oz. (28g) cheddar cheese: Vitamin A 5%, Calcium 20%, Iron 1%, Vitamin D 1%, Vitamin B-12 3%, Magnesium 2%

Throughout both pregnancies, I never really discussed my diet, in particular, with anyone. My providers were all aware, to some extent, that I ate lower carb, but it was never really an issue. I think the clinical measurables (blood sugar levels, ultrasound and NST results, bloodwork) spoke for themselves. There was one instance of ketones in my urine at one appointment, but because my MFM team was knowledgeable enough about the distinction of ketosis vs, ketoacidosis, it was a non-issue.

After delivering my son, I ordered a giant Chef salad from the hospital cafeteria. I swear, it was the most satisfying meal I've ever eaten. Everyone was very surprised I didn't order the burger and fries, though.

-Maria Muccioli, PhD, Diabetes Daily

Supplements

What supplements should you be taking? This of course should be discussed with your OBGYN or MFM, but here are a few that I could recommend:

Prenatal vitamin:

Always important, useful, and a healthy baseline for all pregnancies.

A great prenatal vitamin I've found is **Zahler Prenatal +DHA 300.** It has 2000 IU of Vitamin D3, Folate (5-MTHF rather than folic acid), Methylcobalamin (methylated B12), 300mg of DHA as well as some other cool stuff like Choline.

Vitamin D3:

4000 IU/day-studies have shown that this dose is safe and helps prevent preeclampsia, infection, preterm birth, and other complications.

Folate:

Folic acid is what is typically recommended, but folate is the natural, non-synthetic form. I recommend using L-Methylfolate (5-MTHF). Type 1's many times will be positive for the MTHFR (no that isn't a dirty word) gene mutations, which causes problems with methylation. This form of folate is already methylated, so it's a good idea to use this form just in case (it won't hurt if you don't have the mutations). Folate helps prevent spina bifida and lip/tongue tie. Many doctors are recommending high-dose folic acid/folate, up to 5000 mg per day for diabetics. Check with your doctor on this.

BEST AND WORST FORMS OF MAGNESIUM

Best forms	Worst Forms
Magnesium Glycinate	Magnesium Oxide
Magnesium Chloride	Magnesium Sulfate
Magnesium Malate	(epsom salts)
Magnesium Taurate	Magnesium Aspartate
Magnesium Carbonate	Magnesium Glutamate
Magnesium Citrate*	

*HAS A LAXATIVE EFFECT

Magnesium:

Type ones tend to be low in magnesium already, especially if blood sugars are high. Add to that that our soil is depleted, and our water is filtered. Magnesium has also shown to help prevent preeclampsia. Guess what they give moms who have preeclampsia? You got it, I.V. magnesium sulfate. So which kind should you take?

Magnesium Glycinate is my favorite form of magnesium, but these are some good choices. Magnesium Citrate may have a laxative effect, which actually could be very helpful during pregnancy.

DHA/EPA:

If your prenatal doesn't include these fatty acids, which are important for baby's developing eyes and brain, you might want to include these. They've also been shown to help prevent preterm labor and lower the risk of preeclampsia. The American Pregnancy Association recommends 300mg of DHA daily. Make sure to get high-quality fish oil. If it smells or tastes fishy, it's likely rancid.

Iron:

Most prenatal vitamins will already have an iron supplement. If you have problems with anemia, your doctor may recommend iron supplements. Ferrous Sulfate is usually prescribed, which can cause constipation (you don't need any more of that) and is hard on the gut all around. Ferrous Gluconate is easier on the tummy. I really like Feosol with Bifera, which is an iron supplement with heme iron, which is absorbed better and is gentler on the tummy. It also can be taken with food (ferrous sulfate can't be taken with food).

Chapter 5: The First 4 Weeks

Highs-The First Symptom

Q: Is it normal for my insulin needs to increase as early as 4 weeks? I've been following Dr B's protocol and had my basals and a1c just where I wanted them (both drifting down nicely). Just found out at 3w5d (haven't even missed my period yet) that I'm pregnant and now my insulin needs have changed out of the blue. I've already upped basals by 60% and I have to take a (what now feels 'significant' compared to a few weeks ago) dose for anything I put into my mouth, even a few bites of grilled chicken - I didn't need to dose for that before. Now, my fasting numbers are stuck at 160s (70-90 before)

A: You may have noticed that after you ovulate (around day 14 of your cycle), blood sugars start going up, and keep rising until after your period starts. This varies woman to woman, but it is very common. One of the reasons for this insulin resistance is increased levels of progesterone. This hormone rises after ovulation in preparation for pregnancy and drops after your period starts. Progesterone levels continue to rise until 7 or 8 weeks when the placenta starts to take over, so the first symptom many women see is high blood sugars.

A pregnancy is counted from the first day of your last menstrual period so, when you miss your period, you are considered to be 4 weeks pregnant. Many women have no symptoms at this point other than the highs. Others experience extreme fatigue and sore breasts.

This period of time it is very important to keep blood sugars normal, so knowing your body and spotting a pregnancy right away is key here, as are maintaining normal blood sugars prior to pregnancy. Some of us weren't prepared like we should have been though. Thankfully, my mother taught me to track my ovulation when I was a teenager, so I knew right away that I was pregnant. I had positive results 3 days before my missed period with all three.

Pregnancy Tests

Most women prefer the digital tests for definite confirmation of pregnancy, since they display, 'pregnant' or, 'not pregnant'. The issue with these is that they aren't as sensitive as some of the other tests, and may say, 'not pregnant' when you actually are. In my experience, the most sensitive tests are the ones from the Dollar Tree, or the 88 cent ones from Walmart. It seems counterintuitive, but it's true! These two tests pick up HCG at very low levels. For me, at 3 days before my missed period.

For best results, use first morning urine, and avoid tests with blue dye. The blue dye tests are reported to show false positives, which in most cases, is otherwise rare.

Get on top of it quickly!

The first step is to test blood sugar frequently if you aren't already. We want to test fasting, two hours after your first bite of breakfast, before lunch, two hours post, before dinner, two hours post, before bedtime, and 3am, MINIMUM. Many women test 10x a day or more. If you have the ability to obtain a continuous glucose monitor, this is *highly* recommended for pregnancy.

A continuous glucose monitoring system (CGMS) is a piece of equipment that consists of a sensor (a hair thin piece of wire that goes under your skin and measures the glucose in your interstitial fluid), a transmitter which sends the readings to your receiver or your phone. The two most popular CGMS devices are **Dexcom** and **Medtronic**, both of which take a reading every 5 minutes. The **Freestyle Libre** is considered a flash glucose monitoring system. You scan your sensor, and a reading pops up on your receiver or phone, but it does not have continuous readouts or alarms/alerts. The **Freestyle Libre 2** has recently become available in the US and I hear the **Freestyle Libre 3** is available in Europe. The Libre 2 features alerts and alarms whereas the original Libre does not. You still have to scan to get a glucose reading, but you don't have to scan to receive the alerts and alarms. I personally tried the original Libre when it first came out and found that it read 20-30mg/dL low (as do the Freestyle meters with me). It would say I was 55mg/dL (3 mmol/L) and I'd be 80mg/dL (4.4 mmol/L). Big difference! I am told the Libre 2 is more accurate, but still reads around 10mg/dL low for some people. Something to keep in mind.

There is also a new implanted CGMS called the **Eversense**. It is surgically implanted in your arm and has to be replaced every 3 months. The Medtronic CGMS is integrated with their insulin pump and the Dexcom is integrated with the Tandem X2 insulin pump. Both pumps have features that suspend your insulin if blood glucose drops below a certain level.

The next step is correcting quickly or preventing excursions in the first place. You will likely find that your insulin needs change right away with pregnancy and your insulin to carb ratio, sensitivity and basal needs will need to be adjusted frequently. Some people don't feel comfortable making their own changes and rely on an endo or CDE which is fine, but don't let yourself run high for an extended period. Don't wait until your next appointment if it is days or weeks away. Call and explain the situation.

I had a CDE (her name is Olivia Woods, and she is the one who inspired me to become a CDE so I could help pregnant women like myself!) helping me adjust my pump settings who called every two days with my first pregnancy, and I made all adjustments myself with my second two. Insulin needs change very frequently during pregnancy. I sometimes was making changes as often as every day or two.

Insulin Pumps

Insulin pumps are a popular choice for type 1's and I have done my share of pumping. Dr. Bernstein is not a fan of pumping, and his reasons are valid. His main concern is scar tissue. I am a testament to that. After pumping for close to 20 years and using my abdomen repeatedly, I ended up with scar tissue, and horrible absorption in my abdomen. I had to stop pumping and I didn't use my abdomen for more than a year to give it a break.

If you do pump, rotating sites is *IMPERATIVE*. While I'm not a huge fan of the Omnipod, it does give the opportunity for more sites that tubed pumps don't. Make sure you are changing out your sites every 3 days at the very most. Many find the need to change every two days, especially if using the steel cannulas, which are what I use when pumping to avoid kinked cannulas.

That brings me to my next point. Cannulas can get bent. Tubing can snap. Air can get in your line. The pump itself can malfunction, and since you aren't using long-acting insulin, you can go into DKA rapidly if you aren't checking blood sugars meticulously (or using cgm). I had an instance of mild DKA during my last pregnancy due to my pod coming loose and the cannula partially coming out. I went to bed and woke up with 300mg/dL (16.6mmol/L) blood sugars, nausea, and very high ketones. This required hospitalization and my baby wasn't looking too good for a while. This is definitely something to keep in mind as well. Pumps fail.

There are some benefits to pumping, however. You can give tiny corrections (such as 0.2 units to correct a 110mg/dL to target), multiple basal rates to tailor to your unique insulin needs throughout the day and night, the bolus calculator is super helpful (though the Inpen smart insulin pen offers this as well), and you can give multiple boluses without having to inject each time. The fact that you are using rapid acting insulin is also a benefit when you need to make rapid basal changes. With very long-acting basal insulin like Tresiba, it can take a while to see a change take effect. I found the pump to be a godsend while pregnant. I can take it or leave it otherwise.

> Starting with the first trimester, I had to make some adjustments for meal-time insulin doses since I wasn't eating the same foods as usual due to my aversions. I quickly learned the new dosing and really didn't have many problems. Once I switched back to real food, I re-adjusted my mealtime insulin again. My mealtime doses stayed pretty much the same until week 30 or so, and then they gradually increased until week 38. During the first trimester, I did have some difficulty with blood sugars in the mornings during which I would often shoot up to 150 right after waking up. This was not every day so it was difficult to predict but I was able to take some Humalog when waking and I would have Sweet Tarts if I started going low later. My correction factor gradually increased (needed more per dose) throughout the pregnancy.

> I relied on my Dexcom majorly to determine my needed adjustments to my basal. Around week 10, I noticed my numbers were overall higher and I increased my basal by about 20%. This ended up happening every few weeks throughout the pregnancy. Sometimes my increases were more or less. Starting in week 30, it was more like 10-30% every week. By the time I delivered, I was using 3.5x the total daily insulin as pre-pregnancy!

> Despite the constant changes, I rarely had numbers above a 120. I would dose a correction if I were over a 90. My A1C stayed around a 4.8 throughout my pregnancy according to my Dexcom and Sugar Mate app. Note that it tested anywhere from a 4.6 to a 5.3 at the doctor's office, but my apps showed me there was never any variation week to week. My lines were SO FLAT on my Dexcom.

> On a side note, I use Multiple Daily Injections (MDI). I have never had success with pumps and don't plan on trying one again for a very long time.

> -Olivia

Hybrid Closed Loops have become popular in the last few years. What is a hybrid closed loop you ask? It is a setup where you have an insulin pump and a continuous glucose monitor. The pump receives the sensor glucose readings and adjusts insulin based on these readings.

Currently **Medtronic** has the **630g** which is not a hybrid closed loop, the **670g** and the **770g** which has just been released. The **780g** is set to be released this year (2021). The 670g features automode, which attempts to keep blood glucose in a target range by adjusting basal when blood sugar is rising and suspending the pump when blood sugar is dropping.

Unfortunately, the current target of 120mg/dL (6.7mmol/L) is too high for pregnancy, and too high for those of us who target normal blood sugars. I'm told the 780g will have a lower target of 100mg/dL which is better, but still too high in my opinion. When you're targeting 60-95mg/dL, that just won't work. The suspend on low and suspend before low features seem to result in rebound highs later in my experience as well. The current 770g combines the hardware of the 780g with the algorithm of the 670g. They all use the Guardian sensor, which requires 2 calibrations per day and can be worn for 7 days. Some folks are using older Medtronic models such as the Paradigm 722 for DIY looping. This can't be done with the newer pumps, however.

The **Tandem X2** pump comes with two possible features, **Basal IQ**, and **Control IQ**. With Basal IQ, "If the glucose level is predicted to be less than 80 mg/dL, or if a CGM reading falls below 70 mg/dL, insulin delivery is suspended." This can be very helpful in avoiding nighttime hypoglycemia. In my experience the insulin suspension is not as long as Medtronic and I didn't see the rebound highs.

Control IQ is a hybrid closed loop that has a target range of 112.5 to 165mg/dL (6.2-9.1 mmol/L). Sleep mode is 112.5mg/dL to 120mg/dL (6.2-6.9 mmol/L) which again, is too high for pregnancy (and for me). It suspends the pump when blood sugar drops below 70mg/dL or is predicted to drop below 70mg/dL (dropping rapidly). If your blood sugars are wildly fluctuating and/or you aren't aiming for super tight control, this may be an option for you. Some people have reported, "hacking" CI by running the pump in sleep mode 24/7, (known in the Tandem world as, "sleeping beauties") and calibrating their Dexcom to read higher, so when the pump thinks they are say, 115 mg/dL (6.4mmol/L), they are actually 85 mg/dL (4.7 mmol/L) and are getting great results. This is obviously not something that is FDA approved and at your own risk. The Tandem pump also allows very tiny basal increments of 0.001 so adjustments can be completely customized and work well with children and insulin sensitive individuals. Another great feature of Tandem pumps is that you can upgrade the firmware remotely, without the need of a new pump.

The **Omnipod** is a tubeless waterproof insulin pump/patch. **Omnipod Dash** is Omnipod's latest release. It has a Smart Phone-like touch screen PDM and a mobile app called Omnipod VIEW (only for iOS currently). It uses Bluetooth technology instead of RF (radio frequency) so is not loopable like the original Omnipod. The original Omnipod uses **Freestyle** strips for readings (which in my experience read low) whereas the Dash uses **Contour**. To my knowledge, the Contour meters are the most accurate and are what I use and recommend to my clients. Anecdotally, I had a client, who by blood glucose average should have had an a1c of around 4.8%, but she was closer to 5.8%. I asked what meter she was using and it was Freestyle. I switched her to a Contour and within a few weeks, her a1c was down to 4.8%.

The Dash can receive remote boluses up to 50 feet away, whereas the original Omnipod PDM has to be within 5 ft. The Dash also allows 0 basal rates, so if you are to the point in pregnancy where you're using a ton of insulin and having to change your set constantly, you could go "untethered" and use basal insulin for basal and just use the pump for boluses. The Omnipod is not currently integrated with cgm, but the upcoming version, **Omnipod 5 (formerly named Horizon)** will be integrated with the **Freestyle Libre 2**. This system is a hybrid closed loop and is set to be released in 2021.

I personally had issues with the Omnipod as the basal increments of 0.05 were too big. 0.05 sounds like a really small number, but the difference between say, 0.7 units per hour and 0.75 units per hour were the difference between high blood sugars and low blood sugars. I needed something in between.

There is a newer, more unknown pump called the **DANA RS** pump that was specifically made for DIY looping and includes 2-way communication capabilities between the pump and a smartphone app without the need for an extra piece of equipment (Rileylink) that typically allows pumps and phones to communicate. It is lightweight and is lower costing than other comparable insulin pumps. It can be used with a smart-phone app to change settings, basal rates, and to

DON'T LEAVE HOME WITHOUT YOUR PANCREAS!

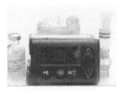

ALWAYS CARRY WITH YOU:
- NOVOLOG/HUMALOG/ADMELOG VIAL OR PEN, SYRINGES OR PEN NEEDLES
- LANTUS/LEVEMIR/TRESIBA VIAL OR PEN IF MDI
- GLUCOSE METER & STRIPS, EXTRA CGM SENSOR
- EXTRA INFUSION SETS, RESERVOIRS, AND BATTERY IF PUMPING
- A COPY OF YOUR BASAL RATES, INSULIN TO CARB RATIO AND CORRECTION FACTOR IF PUMPING
- GLUCOSE TABS, LIQUID GLUCOSE, SMARTIES, SPREE OR BOTTLE ROCKETS FOR LOWS

IF PUMP FAILS:
- TEST BG AND KETONES. GIVE CORRECTION OF RAPID ACTING INSULIN IMMEDIATELY. IF KETONES ARE HIGH, INCREASE THE CORRECTION BY 50%.
- IF NEW PUMP WILL ARRIVE THE SAME DAY, INJECT AT LEAST EVERY 3 HOURS TO CORRECT AND MAKE UP FOR LOST BASAL. IF NEW PUMP WILL NOT ARRIVE THE SAME DAY, GIVE A SHOT OF LEVEMIR/LANTUS/TRESIBA EQUAL TO YOUR DAILY TOTAL DOSE OF BASAL INSULIN PLUS 10%.

GritCDE

This infographic is adapted from a handout we used in Dr. Michele Zerah's endocrine clinic. The original author is unknown.

bolus remotely. Like the Tandem pumps, it's firmware can be updated remotely, and you don't need to get a whole new pump for upgrades.

Pumping has pros and cons and is a completely personal decision. You can get the *same* great results with multiple daily injections. A pump is *not* a necessity for a healthy pregnancy.

Looping and Pregnancy

Looping is a 'do it yourself' version of a hybrid closed loop. I personally have a bit of experience with DIY looping. It can be a great tool. There are a few applications out there including LOOP, Android APS and Open APS. You have to source a loopable pump (I used an old Medtronic 722), and depending on which pump, you may need a device called a Rileylink that allows your phone to talk to your pump (converts RF frequency to Bluetooth). You also have to build the app yourself. There are step-by-step instructions online, so you don't have to be a programmer or anything to build it. The great thing about DIY looping is that you can set your own targets. I set mine to 83 mg/dL (remember Medtronic and Tandem have higher targets than would work for pregnancy). Looping is *not* FDA approved and is completely at your own risk, but many people get amazing results with it. A friend of mine looped during 2 of her pregnancies and I asked her to share her story.

> I've had two very healthy Loop babies, and I'd like to tell you a little about how I did it.
>
> I started using Loop on an old Medtronic 523 pump at the beginning of April 2017. I found out I was pregnant a few days later, so I quickly did some research and worked to gain even tighter control of my blood sugars. The more stories I read, the more anxious I became about outcomes. It seemed like every pregnant woman with type 1 diabetes (T1D) had complications, they all had big babies, and most pregnancies ended in a C-section. Diabetes had never held me back yet, and I wanted to experience as normal of a pregnancy as possible, including a vaginal delivery of a healthy baby. I had successfully completed two marathons just five years earlier, and I was determined to master the challenge of being pregnant with T1D.
>
> It took work, that's for sure. Prior to Loop, I had checked my blood sugar between 12-14 times per day and micromanaged my blood sugars. My A1C ranged from 6.1-6.5%. Once I started on Loop and started to figure out how it worked, I was able to achieve A1Cs between 5.2-5.7%, and with less micromanagement. However, pregnancy required a whole new level of vigilance, as my insulin needs changed fairly often. Throughout pregnancy, I did not eat low carb, but having seen the benefits of a Paleo style approach from completing a Whole 30, I knew a Paleo approach would help me a lot.

I learned to pre-bolus (give insulin and wait between 20-60 minutes before eating), and I learned to fine-tune my settings, sometimes as frequently as every few days.

I'd like to take a little time to explain Loop for those who are unfamiliar. It's an app that runs on an iPhone, and it's based on years of work from numerous individuals who got tired of waiting for the industry to come up with a solution that would better manage blood sugars in people who are insulin dependent. It's a do-it-yourself (DIY) approach that requires a certain level of technical bravery, as you have to install your own app on your iPhone; you cannot download the app from the Apple Store. But when you get Loop installed and set up properly, it can be amazing! The app integrates data from a continuous glucose monitor, a pump, and settings in the app to always be calculating (every 5 minutes) where the blood sugar is ultimately going to end up. The app then adjusts basal rates (and in some versions, administers micro-boluses) to try to avoid lows and highs. The major lesson I learned during pregnancy: if Loop isn't able to get you to your target, then some of your settings are off.

Because I had never experienced pregnancy with T1D before, I reached out to a friend of mine who is a coach for people with T1D. She helped me to learn pregnancy with T1D, and I helped her to learn Loop. Together, we achieved some amazing results.

With my first pregnancy, I was induced at 36W4D due to a mild case of cholestasis (an issue with the mom's liver that can increase the risk of stillbirth after 37 weeks). The obstetrician (OB) came in during the induction, cocky as ever, and declared that I was going to have an enormous baby. My oldest was born vaginally at 36W6D, after 40+ hours of labor, and she was 6 pounds and 13 ounces—not huge by any stretch! She was healthy and did not need NICU time due to blood sugar issues. How I enjoyed proving that OB wrong!

By the time I found out I was pregnant again in May 2020, I knew Loop fairly well. I did a lot of research and decided to set tight targets for myself—between 65-120mg/dL—based on research I read from Allison Herschede, my friend who coached me through the first pregnancy, and Dr. Lois Jovanovich. I know we all experience a fairly heavy load of guilt through a pregnancy with T1D, and people encouraged me to be kind to myself and to lighten up on my expectations; they thought a target range that tight was too hard to achieve. But I wanted a healthy baby and a healthy me. I felt like I did not need a wider target range just because some organizations "allowed" patients with T1D to experience blood sugars up to 140mg/dL. I felt like I could handle a tighter range, and I was willing to do some work to achieve that. During my second pregnancy I was able to attain A1Cs between 4.7-5.2%.

I wanted, more than anything, to go into labor on my own, but during the last few weeks of pregnancy, my maternal fetal medicine (MFM) team (high risk OB healthcare providers) discovered that I had a mild case of polyhydramnios (extra amniotic fluid). I had worked so hard to achieve excellent blood sugars, and I ended up with a complication that is so common to women with T1D! I felt judged, and like I had failed. Even though I had worked so incredibly hard, it felt like my efforts were inadequate. I experienced lots of contractions prior to my due date, but none of them started labor. As my MFM team suggested, I was induced between 39 and 40 weeks. Wouldn't you know, during the induction, that same cocky OB came in to see me. "Why haven't you delivered yet?" he wanted to know. "What do you mean?" I asked. "You should have given birth long before now," he declared. I explained the recommendations of my MFM team, based on the latest research, to which he replied, "All you're doing by waiting is making that baby even bigger, and harder for me to deliver." It made me angry. He claimed my baby girl would be well over 9 ½ pounds. She was born vaginally, with no blood sugar complications, at 7 pounds and 14 ounces—again, not huge by any stretch. And oh, how I enjoyed proving that OB wrong!

But I don't want to be defined by what people say I cannot do. I feel immensely proud of the work I did to achieve healthy pregnancies, despite having had T1D since 1993. I grew up in a world that knew T1D because of the movie Steel Magnolias, and for years, I lived in fear of not being able to have my own children. But I had two healthy children, both born vaginally with normal birth weights—and the complications I experienced In pregnancy could have been experienced by anyone, not just those with T1D. I am saddened by how many of us feel the need to justify, defend, and explain ourselves. However, I am incredibly thankful to have been surrounded by people who believed in me and helped me to succeed. I cannot express how deeply grateful I am for Loop and for what it enabled me to achieve; and I am so lucky to know and be supported by people like Allison who are working to help people achieve healthy pregnancies with T1D.

-Michelle Herman

Michelle also runs a Facebook group called DIY Looping and Pregnancy if you would like more information.

Pregnancy Targets

Target blood glucose depends on your doctor, but the most common targets are 60-95mg/dL (3.3-5.2 mmol/L) fasting (some doctors will just say less than 95mg/dL (5.2mmol/L) and less than 120mg/dL (6.6 mmol/L) post meal. This sounds impossible, but when another life is at stake, you find the wherewithal and make it possible. Nobody is perfect and you will have highs and lows, but we want to minimize them.

*2021 ADA guidelines for pregnancy have changed the targets to 70-95mg/dL fasting, less than 140mg/dL 1 hour post meal and less than 120mg/dL 2 hours post meal. I still tend to side with the lower targets as they mirror the blood sugars of non-diabetic pregnant women, but I think the fear of hypoglycemia (and the lawsuits that could go with that) has sparked this change.

If fasting blood sugar is higher than 95 (5.2), you likely need more basal insulin. If you're spiking higher than 120 (6.6) post meal, you likely need more meal-time insulin.

Pre-bolusing is mandatory. I like to bolus (mealtime insulin or correction dose) at least 15 minutes before the meal. In pregnancy, sometimes it is necessary to bolus as early as 45 minutes before eating. It's all trial and error. If you are spiking really high (200 mg/dL (11 mmol/L) or more), don't wait to make a correction. There is still active insulin on board, but that insulin is already taken up by the food. If you are very high two hours post-meal, you likely aren't going to come down on your own. I personally correct right away with micro-boluses.

Making Doctor's Appointments

You'll likely want to let your primary care doctor know right away when you find out you are pregnant. You will need a referral to an OBGYN if you don't already have one. If you do, go ahead, and give them a call. Some want to wait until 8 or 9 weeks for the first visit, but my doctors usually wanted to see me right away. They will most likely refer you to a high-risk pregnancy doctor (MFM or perinatologist).

You'll also want to give your endocrinologist a call and let them know. They'll probably want to see you right away as target a1c for pregnancy is lower than when you are trying to conceive. Target a1c for ttc (trying to conceive) is less than 7%. Target for pregnancy is less than 6%. A baseline eye exam with your ophthalmologist is also recommended as pre-existing retinopathy can worsen in pregnancy. I was seen once each trimester.

During pregnancy, you will feel like you *live* at the doctor. If you work, you'll need to make arrangements with your boss for your appointments. You'll likely be seen once a month by your OB or MFM until 28 weeks, then every two weeks until 32 weeks, once a week until 36 weeks, and twice a week until delivery. Your endo will probably want to see you at least once a month.

Excerpt from Allison's Pregnancy Blog

Had a positive HPT 2nights ago. I've since gone through about 5 tests lol. Have to be sure! I called my primary care doc yesterday and was seen immediately. Had blood drawn, and my HCG is supposedly good.

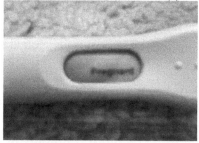

By LMP (last menstrual period) I should only be 3w5d but I'm pretty sure I'm closer to 5 weeks. I'm already experiencing symptoms. Blood sugars are crazy. Fought 200-300's all day Tue, yesterday ranged from 85-180 which isn't quite as bad but not where I want to be.

Today was 160 fasting and 140 2 hours post, which is definitely unacceptable, so I'm gonna have to tweak my basals.

The doctor is referring me to high-risk OB which I do not want. I'm looking into midwives in Savannah, but I doubt they'll take me as "high risk" as I am. I'd like this pregnancy to be as low intervention as possible. I know this is unlikely since I am a T1D with 2 prior cesareans.

Chapter 6: Weeks 4-8

Insulin Needs; "The Lows"

Q: I'm 6w4d and have been dealing with nasty high blood sugars. Last night I suddenly started being constantly low. I'm anxious that I may not be pregnant anymore. Could this be a thing or am I just over-stressing?

A: As previously explained, insulin needs will likely go up until around 6-8 weeks. At this point, it is very common to see a precipitous drop in insulin needs. I called this period, "the lows". I had to keep dropping my insulin and was constantly treating hypos. Some women start making some insulin again during this point in pregnancy. Another reason for this is that progesterone that went up at the very beginning of your pregnancy, causing all those highs, suddenly drops as the placenta starts taking over.

You'll want to keep plenty of glucose or dextrose-based candies on hand during the period of time. Stash it everywhere. Always have a Glucagon emergency kit on hand and make sure your loved ones know how to use it. Eli Lilly recently released a nasal Glucagon. Talk to your doctor about its use in pregnancy. Glucagon does not cross the placenta.

Do Lows Hurt the Baby?

In most cases, no, unless you are low enough that you yourself are harmed (to the point of having a seizure or passing out) or if blood sugar is *very* low for many hours. Baby gets a steady stream of glucose from your bloodstream through the placenta regardless of your blood sugar, even to your detriment. If you have glucose in your bloodstream, the baby will get it. Insulin does not cross the placenta in any appreciable amount.

. . .

We want to avoid lows, of course, Just try to minimize them and correct as quickly as possible. Following Dr. Bernstein's plan helps minimize hypos greatly. If you are only eating a small amount of carbohydrate, you only need a small amount of insulin, so are far less likely to go hypo. Remember also that 60mg/dL is normal in pregnancy. Non-diabetic pregnant women tend to run in the 60's so even though this was considered low before pregnancy, it is not an emergency!

DO YOU KNOW HOW TO USE GLUCAGON?

Glucagon is used in the emergency case of low-blood sugar when the person is unconscious or cannot swallow. In addition to traditional Glucagon injection kits, there is now nasal powder (Baqsimi) and an emergency Glucagon pen (Gvoke). Both are shelf-stable.

GVOKE

- PULL RED CAP OFF
- PUSH YELLOW END DOWN ON SKIN AND HOLD 5 SECONDS. WINDOW WILL TURN RED.
- ADMINISTER INTO UPPER ARM, ABDOMEN OR THIGH.

TRADITIONAL GLUCAGON

- FLIP OFF THE SEAL FROM THE VIAL.
- REMOVE THE NEEDLE COVER FROM THE SYRINGE. DO NOT REMOVE THE PLASTIC CLIP FROM THE SYRINGE.
- INSERT THE NEEDLE INTO THE RUBBER STOPPER ON THE VIAL, THEN INJECT THE ENTIRE CONTENTS OF THE SYRINGE INTO THE VIAL OF GLUCAGON POWDER
- REMOVE THE SYRINGE FROM THE VIAL, THEN GENTLY SWIRL THE VIAL UNTIL THE LIQUID BECOMES CLEAR.

BAQSIMI

- HOLD DEVICE BETWEEN FINGERS AND THUMB.
- DO NOT PUSH PLUNGER YET.
- INSERT TIP GENTLY UNTIL FINGERS TOUCH THE OUTSIDE OF THE NOSE
- PUSH PLUNGER FIRMLY ALL THE WAY IN. DOSE IS COMPLETE WHEN GREEN LINE DISAPPEARS.

TRADITIONAL GLUCAGON CONT.

- INSERT THE SYRINGE INTO THE VIAL AND SLOWLY WITHDRAW ALL LIQUID. FOR CHILDREN <44LB, WITHDRAW HALF THE LIQUID (0.5 MARK ON SYRINGE).
- INJECT IMMEDIATELY AFTER MIXING INTO BUTTOCK, ARM, OR THIGH THEN WITHDRAW NEEDLE. APPLY LIGHT PRESSURE TO SITE.
- TURN PERSON ON THEIR SIDE.

CALL 911 IMMEDIATELY!

Cramping

Q. I need some reassurance! I'm 5 weeks and 2 days... cramping happens I know but it really freaks me out when it feels like period cramps and not just little twinges! This is my first pregnancy, so I'm paranoid because my a1c is 6.8! My numbers have been staying in the 90s for the majority of the day following parameters my doctor gave me. Is this cramping normal? No bleeding, just cramps...

A. I experienced this with all my babies, and it is super nerve wracking. When it happened with my first, I called my OB and he just laughed and said it's totally normal. It happens due to your uterus expanding and your ligaments stretch. If you're worried you can always get checked, just to give you peace of mind. If you see any bleeding, call your doctor right away.

Leukorrhea

Leukorrhea, or the whitish vaginal discharge seen in pregnancy can actually be one of the first signs of pregnancy. If you were tracking your cervical fluid while trying to conceive, you'll be more aware of this. The discharge is typically milky white and thin and will increase in amount as you go further along in your pregnancy.

There should not be any odor or irritation. Leukorrhea is caused by increased estrogen levels during pregnancy.

Many women find it helpful to wear a panty liner.

If your discharge is thick and cottage cheese like, or if it has a foul smell or you experience burning or itching, let your doctor know right away as you could be experiencing a yeast infection or bacterial vaginosis, which you'll want to treat right away. Women with diabetes are more prone to yeast infections, because the yeast thrives on sugar, so if blood sugars are elevated, yeast infections can result.

Pregnancy also makes women more prone to yeast infections. If you do experience a yeast infection during pregnancy, your doctor will likely prescribe a cream, or advise you to buy one over the counter. Diflucan, the prescription pill for yeast infections, is not typically recommended for pregnancy. Check with your doctor on this.

Morning Sickness

Excerpt from Allison's Pregnancy Blog

7 weeks: *Well the lows kicked in just like they always do. I'm out of glucose, gotta go get some more. I've been up all through the night for the last two nights treating lows. Bumped down the late night basals after just bumping them up with all the highs. Frustrating. I got an at home a1c and I'm down to 6.3, much better than before. I'm afraid of gaining too much weight treating all these lows. My pants are getting uncomfortable. I really wanted to hold off on maternity clothes for a while, but I don't know how long I'm gonna make it. I'm gonna try the rubber band trick and belly band and see how long that lasts me. Morning sickness is still going strong. I cannot wait until my doctor's appt. Definitely need meds. Like with Aidan, the smell of cooking meat makes me gag. This should be interesting.*

This starts right around the same time as the lows, around 7 or 8 weeks for most. We are all different though. Some will start having morning sickness at 5 weeks and others won't get it at all. Some will vomit, and some will only feel nausea. Side note, during pregnancy, nausea was my only symptom of hypoglycemia, so it was vital to check frequently. Morning sickness does tend to exacerbate ketosis (non-pregnant women with morning sickness have ketones), so make sure to stay well hydrated.

If you are following a standard diet, you may find that crackers, toast, or other bland carbs help with the nausea. If you're eating low carb, you'll have to get more creative. There are low-carb crackers that you can purchase, and there are many recipes on Pinterest that use almond flour, coconut flour, oat fiber and the like. Some find bone broth helpful, as well as ginger. I personally had to use medications. I was on **Zofran** and **Phenergan** until 12 weeks with all three of my babies. Many OB's no longer recommend Zofran and now use the medication **Diclegis**. Vitamin B-6 and half a Unisom can also help.

If you are experiencing vomiting and lows, mini-dose glucagon can be used, though glucagon itself can cause vomiting. This could save an ER visit. Shelf stable Glucagon is now available under the trade name GVOKE. Dr. Bernstein recommends having injectable Tigan (Trimethobenzamide) for vomiting as repeated vomiting can quickly lead to dehydration and possible DKA. Zofran oral disintegrating tablets are also good to have on hand if Tigan is not obtainable. Talk to your doctor about the use of Zofran or Tigan during pregnancy.

Make sure you're taking your prenatal vitamin as the baby needs all the nutrients it can get. You might find you need to take it at night due to nausea, or if your doctor says it's ok, you can take it every other day. If the vitamin causes constipation, your doctor may prescribe a stool softener, or a prenatal vitamin without iron if your hemoglobin is good.

Q: Ugh I forgot how awful morning sickness is. I really don't have any appetite, but I find myself only being able to keep down crackers and other starchy foods. Any ideas for getting through morning sickness while staying low carb?

A: Salty foods like peanuts and pickles can be helpful. If you must have crackers, make your own low-carb crackers like these:

Recipe: Sesame Cheese Crackers

(from https://beautyandthefoodie.com/sesame-cheese-crackers- low-carb/)

Ingredients:

> ¾ cup almond flour
>
> ½ tbsp sesame seeds
>
> ½ tbsp parmesan cheese
>
> ½ cup grated cheddar cheese, or jack cheese
>
> ⅛ tsp sea salt
>
> 1 XL egg white (separate an egg) 2 tbsp water
>
> ¼ to ½ tsp sea salt (to taste)
>
> ½ tbsp olive oil

Preheat the oven to 350 F.

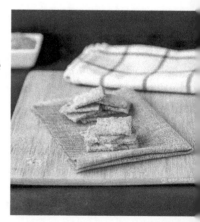

1. In a large mixing bowl, combine the first 7 ingredients, and mix thoroughly, until a dough forms.

2. Remove dough and form into a ball shape and place between 2 large sheets of parchment paper.

3. With a rolling pin, roll dough flat to about an ⅛ to ¼ inch thin.

4. Place both sheets of parchment with the dough onto a baking sheet. Place the baking sheet in the freezer for 10 minutes to firm dough and prevent sticking while peeling off the top layer of paper.

5. Remove from the freezer and gently peel off the top sheet of parchment paper.

6. Using a pizza cutter or knife, slice square shapes into dough.

7. Using a pastry brush, brush the top of the dough with olive oil and sprinkle it with sea salt.

8. Bake for 12 to 16 minutes and turn the broiler on low for one extra minute until browning.

9. Remove crackers from the oven and let cool for 30 minutes or until firm.

You can also buy commercially prepared low-carb crackers, like Flackers or Phat Crackers. Make sure to read ingredients though and make sure there are no no-no ingredients like tapioca starch or arrowroot powder. Many grain-free options are not low-carb.

Other Symptoms

In addition to the nausea, you may experience tenderness in your breasts (I experienced this with #3, but not my first two) and frequent urination (not to be confused with high blood sugar). Fatigue will likely continue. You may experience food aversions. You may also be experiencing bloating and constipation. Make sure you are eating plenty of vegetables (or fruit if you are not very low carb). Coconut oil and magnesium citrate can help with constipation and are safe.

Sweeteners

Since we obviously are not eating sugar, what is the alternative? This list shows the glycemic index of sweeteners. I advise diabetics to avoid sweeteners that are higher than a 1 on the glycemic index. People have reported blood sugar spikes even with a glycemic index of 2.

Which sweeteners are safe for pregnancy? Again, nobody wants to experiment on pregnant women, so there are only a few sweeteners that are *officially* deemed safe for pregnancy. According to the American Pregnancy Association, the following sweeteners are generally recognized as safe for pregnancy:

- Rebaudioside A: (Stevia) Acesulfame Potassium:(Sunett)

- Aspartame (avoid Equal as it contains dextrose)

- Sucralose (avoid Splenda as it contains maltodextrin, which is higher on the glycemic index than sugar!) Liquid Sucralose is good.

- Monk fruit extract is also recognized by the FDA as, "generally safe" for pregnancy. Many mamas have reported good results with erythritol, and I used it personally during pregnancy, but it is not officially approved for pregnancy. Others have had good results with allulose. Discuss the use of sweeteners with your doctor and decide what works best for you.

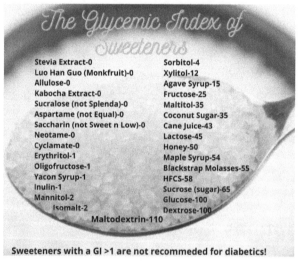

The Glycemic Index of Sweeteners

Stevia Extract-0	Sorbitol-4
Luo Han Guo (Monkfruit)-0	Xylitol-12
Allulose-0	Agave Syrup-15
Kabocha Extract-0	Fructose-25
Sucralose (not Splenda)-0	Maltitol-35
Aspartame (not Equal)-0	Coconut Sugar-35
Saccharin (not Sweet n Low)-0	Cane Juice-43
Neotame-0	Lactose-45
Cyclamate-0	Honey-50
Erythritol-1	Maple Syrup-54
Oligofructose-1	Blackstrap Molasses-55
Yacon Syrup-1	HFCS-58
Inulin-1	Sucrose (sugar)-65
Mannitol-2	Glucose-100
Isomalt-2	Dextrose-100
Maltodextrin-110	

Sweeteners with a GI >1 are not recommeded for diabetics!

Q: I'm 7 weeks and my last A1C was a 6.6%. I'm working really hard to eat low carb, but I've been having a strong meat aversion and nothing seems to help except a little bread sometimes. What should I do?

A: I had a meat aversion with all my babies. You'll need to get your protein from other sources. A whey protein shake can be good (make sure to get unflavored with as few carbs as possible) or you can try full-fat yogurt (unsweetened), Fairlife Milk (lactose has been removed, thus lowering the carbs to 6g), cheese, eggs, and nuts. If you really want bread, there are low-carb bread recipes online, or you can order premade low carb bread made from almond flour, like Fox Hill Kitchens bagels or Smart Buns.

First OB Appointment

Excerpt from Allison's Pregnancy Blog

I had my OB registration appt. They took around 10 vials of blood (12 tests). I was supposed to go today for them to determine if they are keeping me or sending me to the Perinatologist, but the nurse says, "undress from the waist down" and hands me a sheet. Great, I have Aidan with me. The Dr. comes in and says that he wants to do an ultrasound to date the pregnancy and would go ahead and do my Pap Smear as well. Fun times. So, we saw and heard the heartbeat which was around 150 bpm.

The doc is sending me to the perinatologist even though I pretty much begged him to let me stay. He was all for VBAC, acknowledged that ACOG has lowered their restrictions and agreed with me about waiting until 39 weeks (to induce). He said I was up on my info and that inducing early is an outdated practice based on old data. I'm sure I'll have no such luck with the peri.

Most women will have their first OB or MFM appointment during this period. With my first two babies I was seen around 6 weeks and with number 3 I was seen at 8 weeks. You'll likely have a urine sample taken, a lot of blood drawn for various tests, as well as your pap smear, pelvic exam, and many doctors will do a dating ultrasound at this point. This ultrasound will be transvaginal as an abdominal ultrasound won't usually show anything this early. The ultrasound tech will insert a wand into your vagina (don't worry, it isn't painful) to get a clearer view of the baby on the ultrasound.

We were able to see a heartbeat at 6 weeks with #1 and at 5w6days with #2 (I wasn't seen until 8 weeks with #3). When seen this early the heartbeat tends to be lower, so don't worry if it's in the low 100's to 120's. If they can't see the heartbeat this early, they'll likely have you come back at a later period to establish if the pregnancy is viable.

They may see a fetal pole or gestational sac if the heartbeat isn't seen yet.

A urine sample will be taken at every OB visit to look for sugar, protein, as well as ketones (we talked about those earlier), bacteria or blood, which can indicate a urinary tract infection. Many OB's screen for Group B strep in the urine on the first visit as well. Group B strep is a bacterium that can be normally present in a healthy woman's vagina but can be harmful to baby if delivered vaginally. If you are positive, no worries, you'll just be given a dose of antibiotics when labor starts. You will normally be screened for this around 35 weeks of pregnancy with a vaginal swab.

Using a Midwife

It is rare to find a midwife who will take on a type one diabetic (or an insulin dependent type 2 for that matter). We are just considered too, 'high risk'. Occasionally you will find one and if you are able to, take full advantage. Midwives tend to be much more hands-off; interventions are much lower, your risk of Cesarean drops tremendously, and you are more likely to be able to have a water birth, use alternative positions, and overall a much more natural birthing experience. Midwives also tend to let you go full-term if your blood sugar control is tight.

Some midwives work in clinics alongside OBGYN's, so this is a much more likely option for you. My MFM doctor had a midwife who I would see in between visits with him. She championed for my VBAC (vaginal birth after cesarean) and helped convince the doctor to let me go to 40 or 41 weeks.

> My tight control definitely affected my MW's decision to accept me as a patient. They believe completely in supporting women in natural births and use medical interventions only as necessary. When MFM pushed hard for early induction, they supported my decision to wait on the baby (based on my a1c, their size estimates and the fact that I had already successfully vaginally birthed a large baby). We reviewed together the techniques they might use if we encountered shoulder dystocia during labor.
>
> Thankfully, labor started on its own & baby was delivered within minutes of entering the l&d room. (Two more natural births after that- with supportive MWs overseeing my ob. care.)
>
> -Rachel Fontenault

HCG (Human Chorionic Gonadotropin)

HCG is the pregnancy hormone. It's the hormone that is tested when you do a urine test or if your doctor orders a blood test. There are 2 types of blood tests for HCG: qualitative and quantitative. A **qualitative** test also known as gives a 'pregnant' or, 'not pregnant' result. It's just like a urine test, except they put a drop of the serum your spun down blood on the test rather than urine. I used to work as a medical assistant in two OBGYN offices before I was a nurse, and we used the exact same tests that you use at home, *except* they weren't as sensitive! They didn't show a positive result until HCG levels reached 100mIu/mL, whereas those dollar store tests showed in a study to be 100% accurate at 25mIu/mL.

A **quantitative** test, also known as, 'beta HCG', shows the actual level of HCG in your blood. With my first pregnancy, my initial HCG value came back at 32 mIu/mL at 3 days before my missed period. A qualitative test would have shown negative.

Miscarriage

Miscarriage is every mama's worst nightmare (after stillbirth), but unfortunately, sometimes it just happens. It's actually more common than one might think.

Sometimes the pregnancy just isn't viable, and your body knows this. Diabetes (think high blood sugars) can increase the risk of miscarriage, but it doesn't happen from one or two (or 5) highs. It happens with *prolonged* highs. I had a t1 patient when I worked as a medical assistant in an OB GYN clinic. She was running 400mg/dL all day long, and sadly miscarried. This is why it is so important to get blood sugars in check *before* becoming pregnant.

Obviously, we aren't all going to do that, so getting them under control as quickly as possible is essential.

Miscarriage is a huge loss. Take the time to mourn your pregnancy. Even if you were very early, it can be just as painful as a late-term loss. Reach out to friends and family for support. Many have been where you are, even if you don't realize it now.

> *I will preface this by saying that I feel extremely fortunate. In four years, I have had two very healthy pregnancies and children and did not experience any health complications related to diabetes for myself or my two babies. I did experience multiple pregnancy losses, unrelated to diabetes. Both of my two living children are "rainbow babies". Pregnancy carries inherent risks for all women, but as all mothers will undoubtedly tell you: the high risk is worth the great rewards.*
>
> -Maria Muccioli, PhD, Diabetes Daily

Chapter 7: Weeks 9-12

Symptoms

If you are experiencing morning sickness, it usually continues until the second trimester (13 weeks) at least. Constipation will likely continue, as well as the fatigue, and breast tenderness. You'll likely keep having the food aversions as well. Make sure you are getting good nutrition during this time, as the placenta takes over around 10 weeks and what you eat goes to the baby.

Insulin Needs

Insulin needs tend to stay lower (though again, everyone is different). Continue to adjust as needed and correct highs quickly. Treat lows right away, and always have something on hand to treat a hypo. If your insulin need start climbing, make sure to change your ratios/correction factor etc., or let your endo/CDE know so they can make changes. Don't wait!

After the placenta has taken over around 10 weeks, you might notice more highs in the morning. In addition to the Dawn Phenomenon and "Feet on the Floor" (cortisol awakening response; a rise in blood sugar due to stress hormones from waking) that you might already be familiar with, a placental hormone known as human placental lactogen or human chorionic somatomammotropin causes insulin resistance in the morning. Due to this you'll want to avoid fruit altogether for breakfast, low carb or not, and you'll want to minimize your carb intake in the morning.

You might also need a lower insulin to carb ratio (more meal-time insulin) and lower correction factor (more insulin needed for corrections) in the morning.

If you can't stomach meat and eggs, try a low carb protein shake made with unsweetened almond milk or Fairlife Milk (low carb milk that has had lactose removed). High Key Cereal and Magic Spoon Cereals are low carb cereals that don't spike blood sugars in most people. There are also plenty of low carb cereal and hot cereal recipes here: https://www.pinterest.com/typeonegrit

First Trimester Testing

In addition to your ultrasound and routine blood tests, there is also a blood test to rule out birth defects. Prenatal Cell-Free DNA (cfDNA) is a blood test that analyzes the baby's DNA that goes into Mom's bloodstream through the placenta. This test can tell you if you're at risk for things like Down's Syndrome, Trisomy 13, and Trisomy 18. This test is done around 10 weeks of pregnancy. Bonus-you can also find out the gender! This test is also referred to as NIPT or Non-invasive prenatal testing.

Around 11 weeks, your doctor will likely perform a test called the first trimester combined test, which includes a special ultrasound which measures the nuchal fold (the clear space at the back of the baby's neck), and a blood test that measures specific proteins and hormones. These tests performed together can tell you if your baby is at risk for Down's Syndrome or Trisomy 18. This test can be performed between 11-14 weeks of pregnancy.

Another test that can be performed in early pregnancy is the chorionic villus sampling (CVS)test. This test is more invasive than the others and involves removing a sample of the chorionic villi from the placenta. This can be performed vaginally or through your abdomen. This test can reveal chromosomal abnormalities, but there is a level of risk involved. There is a small chance of miscarriage, of Rh sensitization, and infection. This test is usually done if you have shown to be high risk on the prenatal screening. It is performed around 10 weeks of pregnancy.

Tests for Mom

Baby isn't the only one getting tests and exams. Your doctor will likely want a baseline EKG and/or echocardiogram. You'll be assessed by an ophthalmologist to see if there is pre-existing retinopathy. You'll be screened for kidney problems as well as other complications that can cause problems with pregnancy.

You'll also be having pretty frequent a1c's drawn and perhaps a fructosamine level, which shows more current blood sugar control. You'll see your endo more frequently, likely every 3 weeks or once a month with frequent calls from your diabetes nurse or CDE.

Your thyroid should also be tested as autoimmune thyroid disease (Hashimoto's Thyroiditis) is commonly seen in patients with type 1 diabetes. TSH and Free T4 should be tested, as well as Free T3. TSH is recommended to be lower than

2.5 in pregnancy. Free T3 which is the active thyroid hormone, should be in the upper quartile of the range. According to Dr. Bernstein, Free T3 is the most important thyroid hormone, and it is rarely tested.

Diabetics tend to have suboptimal Free T3, and Dr. Bernstein prescribes T3 (Cytomel). Others have success with natural desiccated thyroid (NDT) which is a prescription thyroid replacement sourced from pigs.

Untreated hypothyroidism even with mildly elevated TSH can cause problems for baby. If you suffer from hypothyroidism, I highly recommend the book, "Stop the Thyroid Madness" by Janie A. Bowthorpe. In my opinion, it's like Dr. Bernstein's book, except for thyroid.

"Sneak Peek" Test

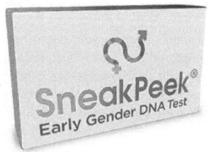

This is a finger stick DNA test that you do at home and mail in. It is offered online for $79. The claim is that it will reveal the gender of your baby as early as 8 weeks and is over 99% effective if done at 8 weeks. You can fast track your results to 72 hours if you pay for the upgrade at $149. To date there are close to 5000 5-star reviews on the accuracy of this test.

Apparently, to get an accurate result, the area where the test is taken should be sanitized and the test should not be taken around any male DNA (even male pets!) Hands should be carefully washed, and you should clean under your fingernails.

Obviously an NIPT test will be more accurate, but this could be a fun thing to try.

CDE/Dietitian Visit

Excerpt from Allison's Pregnancy Blog

I had the dreaded CDE appointment on Wed. I went in there knowing exactly what they were going to say.

30-45g of carbs for breakfast and lunch, 45-60 for dinner and 3 snacks of 15-30g each. Umm, YEAH RIGHT. There is no way! She kept stressing how I NEED carbs right now, my baby NEEDS CARBS. Last time I checked; baby needs GLUCOSE which he will get either way. Carbs or no, my body will produce glucose, and I get all the nutrients I need from meat and vegetables.

She asked if I was testing for ketones with all the lows. I said, "I thought you were supposed to check ketones when HIGH". She says, "no I'm pretty sure it's when you're low" She gets a book and looks it up and is like, "oh yeah I guess you're right". She then proceeded to say that we need to make sure that I am not burning fat for fuel because ketosis is not a healthy state for anyone, pregnant or not. UGGGH. Do some research lady! She also bemoaned the dangers of saturated fat. Sigh. An hour of my life was wasted. Ok, stepping off my soap box.

You'll probably have a consultation with a certified diabetes educator or dietitian which can get dicey if you're following a low-carb diet. Healthcare providers in general are taught the standard nutrition guidelines, which as we know, are totally wrong! It is very possible that your provider will not be on board with a low-carb diet, and if that is the case, you'll have to make the decision whether to follow your doctor, or to go with your gut, and this can be VERY difficult when there is bullying going on. Providers like to play the 'dead baby' card, which is obviously terrifying. Who would want to harm their baby?

I advise you to do your research and educate yourself. Some moms make the decision not to mention diet to their doctor. After all, they are eating meat, vegetables, and healthy fats and are getting better than normal nutrition. Some feel the need to be completely open and there is nothing wrong with that either. They do their research and attempt to educate their provider about the safety of low carb. Sometimes this is effective, but many times it isn't. Remember, this is YOUR body and YOUR baby. The decision is yours.

As you might have guessed, my endo was not on board. He told me I could eat whatever I wanted when not pregnant, but said it was imperative that I eat AT LEAST 100 carbs per day (which is on the low-end for many providers; some want 250g). I had done my research and was convinced that this way of eating was safe for me and my baby, so I continued. My endo and I mutually fired each other mid-pregnancy and I haven't seen an endo since! My MFM doctor was fine with this because my blood sugars were so well-controlled, and the baby looked great on the ultrasounds and monitoring.

Appetite

Q: I'm around 12 weeks pregnant and I'm following Dr. Bernstein's plan. I find I'm feeling super hungry in the late evening or if I wake up during the night. It seems that my body is letting me know I need to eat. I seem to be most insulin sensitive in the late evening, and I know it's super important to keep bg level throughout the night. How do you manage covering bedtime snacks? I'm always scared to go to bed with an active bolus and tend to sleep through alarms. Do you keep the portions small or just stick to protein and no carb for bedtime snacks?

A: Protein promotes satiety. If you find yourself hungry at night, try a snack like meat rolled up with cheese or a spoonful of unsweetened peanut butter. A bedtime snack with carbs is not needed if your basal insulin is accurate. If you find you're dropping overnight, your basal likely needs to be adjusted. Make sure you're getting plenty of protein with your meals and don't worry about the fat that comes along with it. It will keep you full for longer. You can also do a calorie free snack like sugar free jello (choose the one without maltodextrin). Protein snacks will of course need to be covered with insulin.

Chapter 8: Weeks 13-16

Second Trimester

You made it through the first trimester! If you're lucky, the nausea is gone and you are feeling more energy and fewer unpleasant pregnancy symptoms, though you may still have some symptoms like constipation, as the intestinal walls have relaxed. Most women think this trimester is the easiest as the early pregnancy symptoms have gone away, you have more energy, you aren't too big yet and can still breathe! Baby is as big as a peach, bones are forming, intestines are moving into the abdomen from the umbilical cord, and your baby's pancreas is starting to produce its own insulin.

You may find that your clothes are too tight, and that maternity clothes are oh so much more comfortable even if you aren't technically, "showing" yet, though some people are. I definitely was! I swear, I lived in yoga pants during this period. You might still be getting away with the rubber band on your pants trick, but I was not so lucky.

Belly bands, a cloth band that goes around your waist and over your unbuttoned pants are another option to hold off maternity clothes.

Your OB or MFM will likely be able to hear your baby's heartbeat via doppler at this point and will probably start measuring your abdomen (fundal height) at this stage. The doctor or nurse will take a tape measure and measure the distance between your pubic bone and the top of your uterus in centimeters. The number will generally match pretty closely to your weeks of pregnancy and can indicate if the baby is measuring big or small based on this.

From 12 weeks of pregnancy on, you may be advised to take an 81mg baby aspirin every day to help prevent preeclampsia.

Because the baby is making its own insulin at this point, it can already start getting too big (macrosomic) if your blood sugars are high, so continue to be vigilant about blood sugar control. If you aren't getting enough test strips, ask your doctor to write a prescription for more, and to write a prior authorization if necessary.

Insulin Needs

Obviously, your mileage may vary, but most find that insulin needs are still low during this time. Basal adjustments likely still need to be made frequently. If you are still going low, basal insulin needs to go down. If you're going low post meal, your carb ratio needs to go up (less mealtime insulin). If you're seeing highs, it's the other way around of course. Some women find that their blood sugars steadily increase and never have that drop in insulin needs. Keep in touch with your doctor or CDE frequently and make changes as needed. Remember, you don't have to wait until your appointment (and shouldn't).

Q: I've started my second trimester and my blood sugars are in great control, so much so that my insulin needs have gone down significantly! I went from taking a combo of 120 or more units a day of Humalog and Levemir, to 30 a day altogether. Is this normal? I had a scan last week and the baby is fine. Such a sudden drop? I did tweak my carbs and have lowered it to less than 50gms this trimester. Could that be it?

A: Insulin needs tend to go down between 7-18 weeks and cutting carbs will also lower insulin needs, so it's likely both. I haven't found this to be completely accurate, but it's the closest that I've found.

Insulin Requirements during Pregnancy

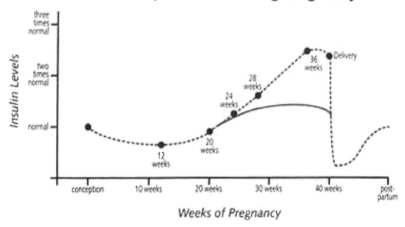

------ = Usual insulin production during pregnancy

——— = Shortage of insulin production during pregnancy with gestational diabetes

You can see it in this graph as well:

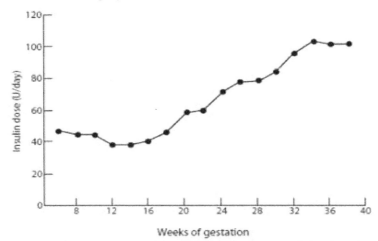

Fig. 1 : Usual Changes in Insulin Requirements in a Patient with Type 1 DM

If you aren't pumping, you will likely need small corrections like ½ a unit or ¼ of a unit to stay in the 60-120 range. There are a few ways to do this on MDI. You can buy syringes with half-unit markings. There is a line for 0.5 units, and you can mark ¼ unit by going between the lines. A second thing you can do is use the **Humalog Luxura**, the **Novo Echo** pens which are reusable pens that you fill with insulin cartridges or the **InPen**, which is a smart pen which has a bolus calculator and other functions of an insulin pump without the pump! These pens go down to 0.5 units. **Pendiq** is a digital insulin pen that goes to 0.1 units but is not widely available.

The last option is diluting. Most doctors are not familiar with diluting and you may get some pushback, but it is a great way to give small doses. Insulin diluent is free from the manufacturer (Eli Lilly or Novo Nordisk) and does not require a prescription. It does however need to be sent to a hospital, clinic, or pharmacy. You can email Eli Lilly for diluent or you can fax a request to Novo Nordisk.

Dr. Bernstein has diluting instructions in his book, and he also has a video on diluting on his YouTube channel Diabetes University. Diluting can be a great tool for children, insulin sensitive adults, or people who need very small doses to target lower numbers, such as in pregnancy!

Screening and Diagnostic Tests

Maternal serum alpha-fetoprotein (MSAFP) and multiple marker screening-this is an optional blood test for birth defects like Down's Syndrome or Spina Bifida. Keep in mind this is a *screening* test rather than a diagnostic test, so if the test shows you are at high risk, this does not mean your baby has the defect, it just means further testing is warranted.

Non-Invasive Prenatal Testing (NIPT) screening or cell free DNA was mentioned in the first trimester tests as it can be done as early as ten weeks. It can also be performed in the second trimester. This test can detect Down's Syndrome up to 99% of the time.

Amniocentesis-this is a diagnostic test that may be recommended if you have an abnormal MSAFP or NIPT, if there is a family history of birth defects or genetic conditions, or if you are over 35 years of age. A thin needle is inserted through your abdomen into your uterus and a sample of amniotic fluid is collected. The test can determine chromosomal abnormalities, or genetic conditions. It is usually performed between 14 and 20 weeks of pregnancy. There is a small chance of miscarriage with an amniocentesis (less than 1%), so this is a personal decision.

Illness

Q: I'm suffering from a bad cold. How do I manage my blood sugars? This is the second time in 3 weeks that I have caught a cold and am having a hard time keeping my numbers down.

Yesterday it took me over 6-7 hours with corrections in between to bring it down to a 97mg/dL. I feel awful because of the cold and slight fever but I really can't do much about it.

P.S I am bolusing extra insulin before meals.

A: I would just keep correcting with fast acting. If it continues more than a few days I might increase basals, but if it is only illness related, just continue with rapid acting. Insulin resistance from illness can come and go quickly, and if you increase basal insulin, it is in your system for a long period of time. If the resistance suddenly disappears, you could have serious hypoglycemia. Ask your doctor which over-the-counter medications are safe to take during pregnancy.

Chapter 9: Weeks 17-20

Increasing Insulin Needs

Q: At how many weeks do you start to see a need for more insulin? I am 17 weeks and have had higher than normal readings the last couple days. Been monitoring because I'm not sure if it's due to travel or the need for more insulin.

A: It is very common to see an increase in insulin needs at this point. Numbers start creeping up and adjustments will need to be made to insulin dosing. Don't be afraid to take more insulin. A non-diabetic mom will be making extra insulin at this point as well. If your insulin needs are still lower at this point, don't worry. This is very individual. I was still running low at 17 weeks.

Dizziness

Remember the old movies where the lady faints, and then finds out she's pregnant? This is likely due to hypotension (low blood pressure) that can happen in pregnancy. Many experience this during the second trimester. Make sure you don't get up too fast, and if you feel light-headed, make sure to drink some water and try eating something salty to bring up your blood pressure. Lying down on your left side can be helpful as well.

Make sure you test your blood sugar when this happens as it could be a result of hypoglycemia. Symptoms of low blood pressure and low blood sugar can be very similar. If you're actually passing out, let your doctor know right away. This is not normal.

Leg Cramps

Q: I've been having severe leg cramps in the middle of the night. From what I can tell, this is pregnancy related. Any ideas on how to stop them?

A: Another second trimester woe that many moms experience is leg cramps. This is often due to an electrolyte deficiency. Low carbers tend to find that they need to supplement electrolytes and diabetics are prone to low magnesium and insulin lowers potassium, so it's important to eat a diet rich in these minerals. You can also make your own electrolyte drink. This is adapted from Dr. Bernstein's recipe in his book.

Leg Cramp Remedy Recipe:

20 oz water (more if this is too salty for you)

1 sugar free flavoring packet (my favorite is Crush Pineapple from Dollar General) or Mio drops

1/2 tsp Himalayan pink salt or **Redmond Real Salt** (regular salt is fine, but I like these for the trace minerals). This provides sodium and chloride.

1/8 tsp **NuSalt** or **Morton Salt Substitute**. This provides potassium. *Note: do not take more than ¼ tsp as too much potassium can cause heart rhythm problems.

200mg Magnesium. I use **Trace Minerals Mega Mag** liquid magnesium. You can also use **Magnesium Calm** powder or Magnesium Citrate from the laxative section (cheapest route). I also found some Magnesium Glycinate Powder on Amazon. Mix well and drink. This recipe is also helpful during morning sickness.

You can also use "Morton's Lite Salt" which is part salt and part potassium. You can use ½ tsp of this instead. If you are looking for a commercially available electrolyte supplement, **LMNT** electrolytes are the best commercially available electrolytes on the market in my opinion.

Anatomy Scan

Excerpt from Allison's Pregnancy Blog

It's a BOY!!! Everything looked great on the scan. They checked everything. We were able to see the chambers of the heart, the brain, kidneys, even the lenses of the eyes!!! I'm still measuring a week ahead, which we expected. Baby was very active. The tech kept commenting on how "busy" he was. He was turning somersaults and kept changing positions and kicking, one time I as well as the tech felt it! We got one 3d shot, but he wasn't in a good position for it, and she said as early as it is, he still looks "skeletor". Afterward Matt and I went to Target and looked at baby stuff. I couldn't resist getting an adorable little romper! Such a great day!!!

Sometime between 18 and 20 weeks, you'll likely have your anatomy scan. This is an in-depth ultrasound that will look at the baby from head to toe to make sure everything is as it should be. The doctor will look at things like your baby's brain, heart, spine, kidneys, eyes and more. You'll also probably get to find out the gender if you haven't already! This is an exciting time for most moms, though it can be anxiety provoking if you're worried something might be wrong. Just try to relax and enjoy seeing your baby.

Your baby's size will also be estimated based on measurements taken during the ultrasound. You might even get the tech to switch to 4d, though baby can look kind of skeletal looking at this point, so don't freak if so.

Feeling Movement

By this point, a lot of moms have felt movement.

First-time moms might not know what to expect. You may have the feeling of "butterflies" in your lower abdomen or feel like a goldfish is swimming across your lower belly. If your placenta is anterior, or if this is your first baby, you may not be feeling movement yet.

Hypoglycemia Unawareness

Excerpt from Allison's Pregnancy Blog

Had a scary low the other day. Was 36 and felt nothing. The cgm was beeping and I felt fine, so ignored it, but finally did a finger-stick when it said "LOW" and it was indeed below 40. I tend to get hypo unaware during pregnancy and that's always scary, so I really need to get a handle on the lows.

I experienced this with all my pregnancies. The only hypoglycemia symptom I had was nausea, which was very confusing during the period of morning sickness. The Dexcom came in really handy with this. Hypoglycemia unawareness is a big indication for continuous glucose monitoring (as is pregnancy). If you cannot obtain a cgm, it is VITAL to test even more frequently.

Chapter 10: Weeks 21-24

Insulin Resistance

The insulin resistance has really kicked in as I was expecting it to. I've had to increase my basals as well as dropping my insulin to carb ratio (down to 1:3 eek!) and my correction factor. Limiting carbs is making a huge difference this pregnancy as far as my meal doses. With the last two I had to take massive doses to cover my carbs and this really helps. After a couple days of nasty numbers, I am back in the "normal" range.

Q: 22 weeks and I've been battling highs all day. I woke up around 130 & stayed in 180-190 range all day. I've changed my sites out 3 times & have taken so much insulin. What am I doing wrong?

A: You're not doing anything wrong! This insulin resistance is completely normal for this stage of pregnancy. It means your placenta is doing what it's supposed to.

Your insulin needs have just increased. You'll likely need more insulin all around, basal and bolus. Some find that light exercise can help some with this as exercise makes us more sensitive to insulin.

Insulin resistance in pregnancy is caused by hormones. In addition to the increased progesterone and estrogen needed to maintain the pregnancy, you have placental hormones such as Human Placental Lactogen. It is a hormone that helps break down the fats mom eats to get fuel to the baby, and it frees up needed glucose that the baby needs to grow and develop. One of the ways it frees up glucose is by causing insulin resistance in mom, which in a non-diabetic is not a problem as the body will make insulin to compensate, but in a diabetic, you'll start having these raging highs.

This is a super frustrating time as you're obviously doing the best you can, and your numbers just aren't cooperating. You're scared you're hurting your baby and doing everything you can to bring down your blood sugar. Just correct as quickly as possible. IM (intramuscular) Injections can be very helpful as they work more quickly and are out of your system faster. Insulin dose will need to be increased all around and frequently.

IM Injections

This sounds like something scary, but in reality, it's just a shot in the arm or leg. Growing up, my mom always injected my arm shots in the deltoid. That's how we had been taught. We didn't know they were IM (intramuscular). If you've ever injected your thigh, you've almost definitely done an IM as most people don't have fat on their thighs, even if they are overweight. 12.7 mm needles were all that were available so that's what I was used to, and they didn't bother me. I buy the longer needle syringes online over the counter and I order the 3/10 cc syringes with half-unit markings so I can take tiny doses. You can read more about intramuscular shots in Dr. Bernstein's book or on his YouTube channel.

Using IM injections to bring down highs fast!

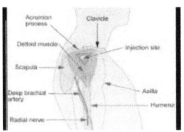

- Dr. Bernstein recommends injecting into the muscle when you need to bring down a high quickly.
- It's recommended to use a 12.7mm insulin needle.
- IM injections are more rapid, but shouldn't be any more potent than a normal shot.
- IM shots are out of the system faster, so you're less likely to stack insulin.
- Dr. B recommends using the deltoid muscle. Spread the skin flat. Don't pinch.
- IM shots are generally painless (unless you hit a nerve)

Gary Scheiner, MS, CDE, author of "Think Like a Pancreas" also has a good article on IM's you can read here: https://diatribe.org/issues/39/thinking-like-a-pancreas.

Fetal Echo

Monday, we had the pedi-cardiologist appt for the fetal echo. It was kind of confusing. The tech doing the echo said they look for thickening in the walls with diabetic mothers, but she didn't see any of that. Then the doctor came in and said everything looked fine. He then went on to say that there was some "mild" thickening and he wanted to re-check in 4 weeks. He finished up by saying everything looked fine.

At some point in the next few weeks, you'll likely be having a fetal echocardiogram. This is a special test that uses ultrasound waves to look closely at your baby's heart. It is usually done by a pediatric cardiologist but can also be done by your MFM. Since diabetics are more prone to having babies with heart defects, this is commonly done for t1's. It takes about an hour but is pretty cool to see all the details of the baby's heart. Don't worry, it's not a scary or painful test, just another ultrasound.

Movement

If you haven't already, you'll almost definitely be feeling fetal movement now, if not hard kicks that can be felt from the outside. I always loved feeling my baby move. It was one of my favorite things about being pregnant. As I got further along, I would put the TV remote on my belly and baby would kick it off!

Alternate Sites

As your belly gets bigger, you might feel uncomfortable injecting or pumping on your abdomen. While there is no way that the needle is long enough to hurt your baby, you may still want to use other sites for comfort. I always liked using my hips/upper butt, and love handle area. I also used my lower back but had a lot of trouble with occlusions there. If you're using an Omnipod, the backs of your arms are a good site.

Colostrum

Q: I'm 23 weeks and today I noticed a few drops of yellowish liquid on my bra. Is this normal?

A: Yes! This fluid is called colostrum and is kind of a "pre-milk". Some refer to it as "liquid gold". It contains valuable antibodies and nutrients for your baby in its first hours/days. Many moms start collecting colostrum in syringes to freeze later in pregnancy to feed to their baby in case of hypoglycemia at birth.

Swelling

Excerpt from Allison's Pregnancy Blog

I'm feeling pretty good. I've been fighting swelling in my ankles, which in the past has started around 20 weeks for me. They were a little swollen one day and since then I've been making sure to take my magnesium and Vitamin D3 regularly, as well as increasing fluids and not eating whole jars of olives ;). My main plan is to stay inside in the air conditioning during this nasty hot weather. I think the magnesium is really helping with bp as well. In the past I've had borderline high bp, but so far, it's stayed around 100/60.

Q: I'm 20 weeks and my ankles are swelling already. Should I be worried?

A: Swollen ankles can be very common in pregnancy, especially if it's hot outside. Drinking a lot of water and keeping your feet up can be helpful. A Magnesium supplement as well as a high protein diet can also help prevent swelling. Compression socks can also be helpful. **Note: you can now buy super cute compression socks on Amazon. No more ugly, old lady, medical looking socks.**

Dr. Gowri Motha, renowned obstetrician and author of "The Gentle Birth Method" says that in addition to hormones, water retention is caused by eating too many carbohydrates. She recommends cutting out wheat and sugar completely as well as avoiding most sweet fruits like bananas, grapes, and mangoes. She also recommends drinking fennel tea to help the body remove retained water.

I personally had horrible swelling with my first two babies. So much that I could not wear regular shoes by the end.

With my low-carb baby, I only had swelling once or twice.

It is important to note that if you have swelling of the hands and face accompanied by headaches or blurred vision, you may be exhibiting signs of preeclampsia, which is a serious condition, so let your doctor know if you have any of these symptoms.

Chapter 11: Weeks 25-28

Braxton Hicks Contractions

Q. I've noticed my belly getting really hard, and then relaxing. It happens more when I've been walking a lot. Are these contractions?

A. Yes, but they aren't labor contractions. They are called Braxton Hicks contractions and they are like, "practice" contractions that tone your uterus and get it ready for labor. Like you said, they can become more frequent if you're very active and can also be brought on by dehydration. If you're having a lot of them, drink some water and lie down on your left side. If you're having 6 or more per hour and they don't stop, give your doctor a call.

I felt BH with my first two starting around 20 weeks and felt them around 12 weeks with number three (of course MFM didn't believe me), but I did some research, and they absolutely happen, most women just don't notice them. If you don't feel any, don't worry, it doesn't mean anything is wrong.

Kick Counts

During this period of time, your doctor may have you start doing kick counts to make sure the baby is moving like it should. Some doctors have moved away from this and say that you know how your baby moves, and if baby isn't moving as expected, to get checked out. If your doctor does have you doing them, he'll likely have you looking for 10 movements per hour. Of course, baby sleeps just like we do, so if baby isn't moving, don't panic! Try drinking a cold glass of water and laying on your left side. If the baby continues to not move like it should, go get checked out.

. . .

Better safe! There are apps for kick counts like "Kick Counter" and "Kickme-Baby Kicks Counter that can be found for free in the app store or play store.

Insulin Resistance is Even Worse!

Almost every t1 mama I have ever encountered says the insulin resistance is the most horrible around 26 weeks. I like to say it, "peaks" at this time, but that is not totally accurate as the resistance continues to increase after this, but it does seem to slow down after this point. There is a reason non-diabetic mamas are checked for gestational diabetes at 26 weeks!

More Tests

While we *do* get to skip the nasty glucose drink for the OGTT (oral glucose tolerance test) at 26-28 weeks, we still get the routine labs like an RPR (rapid plasma regain, a blood test for Syphilis and I know, that made me mad too, but they test everyone), a blood count to test for anemia, and if you are Rh negative, you'll get a Rhogam shot in case your baby has a positive blood type. I am O negative, so I had to get it with all three. You'll get another shot after birth if your baby is positive. Fortunately for me, only one of my babies was positive.

Your doctor may also ask you to do a test called a 24-hour urine. This test is to check for protein in your urine over a 24-hour period. You'll be given a plastic jug and after discarding your first morning urine, you'll collect the rest for 24 hours. You'll want to keep the jug cool. I put mine in an ice chest. This test is an annoyance but can be helpful in diagnosing preeclampsia.

More Frequent Visits

Starting at 28 weeks, you'll probably start seeing your OB/MFM twice a month rather than the once a month up to now. This will increase again at 32 weeks to once a week and to twice a week from 36 weeks on.

Preterm Labor

If you start experiencing cramps in your lower abdomen, persistent Braxton Hicks contractions, persistent lower back pain or leakage of fluids, call your doctor right away. Preterm labor can often be stopped if caught early enough.

There are many reasons for preterm labor. If you have had procedures such as a LEEP (loop electrical excision procedure) or cone biopsy for pre-cancerous cervical cells, you may have a short or "incompetent" cervix. The length of your cervix can be measured via ultrasound if your doctor thinks this may be an issue and your cervix can be stitched closed in a purse string style (a cerclage) until the end of your pregnancy.

Another reason for preterm labor is being pregnant with multiples. Other risk factors are smoking, high blood pressure, history of preterm birth and yes, diabetes.

Preterm labor can happen to any mom though. In the United States, approximately 10% of women experience preterm labor. If you are deemed at risk for preterm labor, your doctor may do a vaginal swab called a fetal fibronectin test. Fetal fibronectin is the "glue" that keeps the amniotic sac attached to your uterine lining. If the amniotic sac starts disconnecting from the lining of the uterus, some of this fetal fibronectin is released and will be around your cervix. This test can predict if you will go into labor within the next two weeks.

There are a few medications that can be used to try and stop preterm labor. One is **magnesium sulfate**, which is also used to treat pre-eclampsia. Magnesium has a muscle relaxing effect and can stop contractions (a good thing to remember if you're supplementing magnesium at the end of your pregnancy). Magnesium Sulfate is given through an I.V. in the hospital and you will be on bed rest. It has some yucky side effects but keeping that baby in there longer is worth any discomfort!

Another medication used to stop labor is **Terbutaline**. Terbutaline is another I.V. medication in a class called betamimetics which relax the uterus and prevent contractions, but it can have some serious risks associated with it. It is only recommended in urgent cases where the risk outweighs the benefit.

Another option is a calcium channel blocker such **Procardia** (nifedipine) which can help relax your uterus and stop preterm contractions. These medications are normally given for high blood pressure and can cause drowsiness and dizziness.

A newer drug called **Makena** can be used to prevent premature labor. It is a synthetic form of progesterone. It is given as a subcutaneous injection and is typically started between 16-20 weeks if you have had a previous preterm baby. It is given weekly until 37 weeks of pregnancy. It will typically be given in your doctor's office, but some doctors will let you do it yourself at home, with an auto-injector especially since you are a t1 who is already giving yourself injections. It is typically given in the back of the arm, so if you wear your cgm sensor in the back of your arm, you may want to use another spot like your upper thigh. You can also ask about giving the injection in your buttocks if you prefer to keep the sensor in your arm. Since we know progesterone can cause insulin resistance, you may have to increase your insulin even more. Makena is not without risks, and as with the other medications, it is a decision based on risk/benefit.

If it looks like your labor may not stop, your doctor may give you an injection of a steroid called Betamethasone to help develop your baby's lungs. Steroids can cause even more insulin resistance, so you may need a good bit more insulin. I had a scary bleeding event at 28 weeks with my second baby and was given this injection. I had to fight high blood sugars for a couple days due to this but helping the baby's lungs develop was definitely the priority.

Premature Baby

If premature labor cannot be stopped, your baby can have a lot of issues, but thankfully, we live in an age where babies as early as 22 weeks can possibly survive (I even saw a story about a 21-week-old baby recently!) Getting to 28 weeks reduces the risks greatly and obviously the farther you can get the better, as baby's brain and lungs are still developing into the late weeks of pregnancy.

T1's are often delivered early due to many different reasons, so preterm birth is more common. As with everything else, keeping blood sugars tightly controlled is paramount.

Late Pregnancy Loss

Sometimes, despite doing everything right, the worst happens. A stillbirth is a loss of pregnancy after 20 weeks. There are many reasons for stillbirth other than diabetes.

Lauren shares her story:

> We had three children while I was diabetic, one in 2012, 2014, and 2018. All of them were hard pregnancies and for two of them I had uncontrolled diabetes. With my daughter in 2018, I had started eating low carb. I found it helped my blood sugar a lot and I was able to take less insulin. She was diagnosed with a heart defect at 30 weeks. I got sent three hours away to Indianapolis with preeclampsia to deliver her in a level IV NICU that could do cardiac surgery if needed. She turned out two have an ASD, VSD, and coarctation of the aorta. Within a year all three had corrected themselves without surgery. This was such a crazy birth we had decided we were done having kids.
>
> Imagine my surprise when I found out I was pregnant again 9 months after her birth. The pregnancy started off well and then I started spotting at 8 weeks. The doctor did an ultrasound, and everything was fine. Two weeks later at work, I started bleeding. Went to the doctor and the baby no longer had a heartbeat. So, January 10th, 2019 I had a D&C. The baby was genetically tested; it was a boy, and he was chromosomally normal. This loss devastated me. It took me 6 months to come out of depression. He

was a total surprise. This started a longing in me for just one more child. So, I began the process again of using lh strips, tons of vitamins, using my Creighton method charting and observations to identify ovulation, post peak progesterone, getting my A1C down to 7. You name it, I tried it to get pregnant.

Finally 16 months after we lost our son, I was pregnant again. I was ecstatic, but cautiously optimistic. I had my HCG and progesterone tested several times and everything looked to be on track. My Napro OB wanted me to start progesterone injections. So I did, starting at 5 weeks 200mg twice a week. They were expensive and they hurt, but it was worth it for my baby. We did the NIPT twice. Both times they came back no result. Turns out it is contraindicated for patients who are obese, have hypertension, and on aspirin therapy.

Made it to our 18-week ultrasound and we found out we were expecting a little girl. Week 19 on Halloween we finally felt safe enough to tell our other children and parents we were expecting. Ten days later I lost my sense of taste. I went and had a rapid Covid test done. I had it. I spent the next 10 days locked in my bedroom. I felt fine overall, just a little tired in the beginning and it hurt to breathe deep for a few days near the end. It went away and I was back to my normal activities. Then I started getting headaches. Went to the hospital expecting them to say my bp was high, but no big deal and send me home. That was not the case. I had developed severe preeclampsia.

They were worried they would have to deliver her at 21 weeks. I was told I would be kept at the hospital until I delivered. My first goal was to get to 22 weeks and then 24. After the first week I was mostly stable. Blood sugars were good, Blood pressure was high but stable. I started thinking about the long haul. My husband brought me my crochet hooks and sewing machine so I could stay busy. He brought me Thanksgiving dinner and I ordered the kids' Christmas gifts online from my hospital bed. Though I had bought and wrapped a ton before I got Covid.

We made it to 24 weeks. I was ecstatic that her chances of survival if I had to be delivered were much better than the two weeks prior. At 24 weeks and 2 days we had a growth scan with my Maternal fetal practitioner. The baby now seemed to have low fluid and IUGR, but her heartbeat was in the 150's and she was very active. Everything looked OK for the time being.

The next day, I swear I felt her kicking at breakfast. The nurse came in to put the monitor on me. For an hour they looked for her. They called in a resident and an ultrasound. Still couldn't find her. Called in an Ultrasound tech and my OB. Found her and there was absolutely no heartbeat. We were all in shock. My MFM, my OB, my nurses...me and my husband. She had been doing so well. I felt anger at God, I felt anger at myself because I was sure the diabetes had done this, even though my A1c was 5.1.

Because of her size the doctors agreed to allow me to be induced and have a VBA3C. They placed laminaria in my cervix and let it ripen overnight. They had seen enough progress that I got put on Pitocin. At about 5:40pm my OB came in to check me. He said it wouldn't be long now and went to change. 5:50pm, I get something wet between my legs. I asked my husband to check it out because I had an epidural and couldn't sit up enough to see. He lifted the sheet. There she was. Out of the birth canal with her cord wrapped twice around her neck. We held her and had a friend who worked for NILMDTS come and take photos.

After three hours the nurses took her away to a cold cot. A sweet nurse named Candace took me to the shower and cleaned me up. I needed that comfort of care. We ate and went to sleep. The next morning they asked if I wanted some more time with her. They rolled her into my room in a bassinet.

She was so cold. It felt like I was cradling a bag of frozen peas not a baby. I couldn't stop staring at her. She was so perfectly formed. Perfect little ears and nose, perfect fingernails and long, long legs. We held her for hours, put a tiny diaper on her, dressed her in tiny clothes, took a million pictures.

Then the funeral home showed up. That was the hardest moment I didn't see coming. This was final. Our baby was going to be returned to ashes. My husband and I cried a lot. My heart hurt so bad I thought it would kill me. We had a funeral a few days later.

Our daughter Margaret Joelle Whalen born December 10th, 2020, will always be with us. I am supposed to be 39 weeks pregnant on Saturday. I am not supposed to be paying off a funeral.

-Lauren Whalen

Losing a child to stillbirth is not something I personally have experience with, but I have seen how painful it is in friends who have lost their babies. Ask the hospital for mementos and take lots of pictures. Lauren mentions NILMDTS: Now I Lay Me Down To Sleep is a charitable organization that will connect you with a local professional photographer, who will come to the hospital to take photos of your infant at no cost. Contact them at https://www.nowilaymedowntosleep.org/

Hold your baby if you want to. Give yourself time to heal. Grieve as long as you need to and don't let anyone tell you how long you're allowed to grieve. Find a support group with other mamas like yourself.

Talk to your doctor about when it's safe to try again. Your body will need to recover from the pregnancy and build back nutrient stores.

Chapter 12: Weeks 29-32

Third Trimester

You are in the home stretch! It's an exciting time, yet it can be miserable as well. All the pregnancy woes are more significant in the third trimester. You'll be seeing the doctor more, having more monitoring (get to see the baby more!), and you'll be taking tons of insulin. Don't panic at the dose. Don't be afraid to use insulin as needed. Take what your body needs. Some mamas are well over 100 units a day at this point, though eating low carb definitely helps with this. I took half the insulin of my previous pregnancies with my low carb baby.

Estimated Fetal Weight

Excerpt from Allison's Pregnancy Blog

30 weeks - After my growth ultrasound, the midwife said that the baby is measuring in the 97th percentile and is huge. Now here is the way I figure it. Diana and Aidan were both 2lb14oz at 28 weeks. The baby is expected to gain around 1/2 lb. a week, so if he is 3lb14oz at 30 weeks, he was around 2lb14oz at 28 weeks just like Diana and Aidan were.

34 weeks - At our appointment yesterday, the estimated weight was 5lb 13 oz, which puts him again in the 97th percentile and 3 weeks ahead. So, going by my counts he's measuring 2 weeks ahead (I'm a week ahead of their due date) and if he gains half a lb. a week, he'll be around 9lb if I go to 40 weeks which means he'd be around 8lb at 38 weeks just like Aidan was (I don't know why I let them get me so worked up!). When the lady was doing my scan, she did the belly first and said, "oh yes chubby tummy, have your blood sugars been bad?" Made me so mad. I told her, "no they've been great!" She looks like she doesn't believe me. Then after she does all the measurements, she says, "oh well in diabetics we usually see just large bellies but he's big everywhere!" I'm like duh, he's just a big baby, he does have a 7 ft tall uncle!

37 weeks - *The monitoring went fine but Adrian measured 8lb14oz! I know the estimates can be off but that is concerning. It seems so unfair that he is so big. I've done so well with my diet and haven't eaten junk, and my blood sugars have been great for the most part.*

At this point in your pregnancy, your OB or MFM may start doing estimated fetal weight via ultrasound. They do this obviously because diabetics tend to have macrosomic (too big) babies. I always hated these as the ultrasound tech always assumed my babies would be big even though I kept my blood sugars tightly controlled. I felt like they used them to make me feel guilty, even though I was doing my best, and my babies had the genetic predisposition to be big. My brother is close to 7 feet tall, the other men in the family are well above 6 feet, my mother was 5'11 and I'm the shortest at 5'9.

The thing about estimated weight is that it is often inaccurate, and doctors tend to induce diabetics early or recommend a cesarean based on these estimates, when they are often very wrong. The day I had my daughter, they estimated she would be 7lb14 oz and she ended up weighing 7lb even. My 3rd was estimated to be greater than 10lb and he was 8lb12 oz (and 21.5 inches to boot, so he was long, and he was big all-around, not just the abdomen as is typically seen in babies of diabetic mothers). Remember you can politely decline these weight estimates and you can refuse an induction or cesarean. It is your body and your baby.

Ultrasound estimation of fetal weight is a highly influential factor in antenatal management, guiding both the timing and mode of delivery of a pregnancy. Although substantial research has investigated the most accurate ultrasound formula for calculating estimated fetal weight, current evidence indicates significant error levels.

> – Julia Milner and Jane Arezina, "The accuracy of ultrasound estimation of fetal weight in comparison to birth weight: A systematic review"

"Regardless of the formula used, the accuracy of the sonographic estimate of the EFW is affected by suboptimal imaging and biological variation. In addition, the accuracy of the sonographic estimate decreases with increasing birth weight and tends to be overestimated in pregnancies suspected of being large for gestational age (LGA) and underestimated in pregnancies with preterm premature rupture of membranes (PPROM) and suspected fetal growth restriction

> - Mark A Curran, M.D., F.A.C.O.G, "Estimation of Fetal Weight and Age"

Now don't get me wrong, diabetics absolutely can and do have macrosomic babies if blood sugars are not tightly controlled, but according to ACOG, macrosomia is NOT an indication for early delivery, and unless the baby is estimated over 4500g, cesarean section is not indicated.

An experienced doctor can estimate better feeling the baby with his hands, than any ultrasound in my opinion. If you do decide to proceed with the estimates, just keep all this in mind, and don't beat yourself up if the baby appears big. Even if the baby *is* big, that doesn't necessarily mean it is your fault and it doesn't necessarily mean you will need a cesarean. Women have delivered 11lb babies naturally with no issues. It all depends on the individual and the doctor.

Pre-bolusing

In the past, you may have only needed to pre-bolus 15 minutes before your meal, but at this point in your pregnancy, you may find that you have to bolus as much as 45min to an hour before eating. Total pain, but necessary.

Monitoring

Many doctors will start NST's (non-stress tests) and BPP's (biophysical profiles) around 32 weeks and your visits will increase to once a week. For a non-stress test, you will have sensors strapped to your belly that track the baby's heart rate and if you are having contractions. You'll be given a button to push when you feel the baby move (some track movement on their own and you don't have to push the button.) If the baby is very active, the test takes 20 minutes. If the baby is sleepy or lazy it could take longer. They are looking for the baby to move, and for its heart rate to increase with movement. If the baby is not moving like they want it to, they might use a "buzzer" on your belly to wake the baby up. It feels like it's zapping the baby, but it's really just noise and doesn't hurt the baby at all.

A biophysical profile is a special ultrasound in which they check for your fluid level, baby's movement, muscle tone and practice breaths. Some doctors will do this in conjunction with a non-stress test, while others will substitute the BPP for the NST since they are already checking movement and heart rate.

It can be a pain to have so many appointments but use this time to relax and take a break. It's also fun to see your baby so often.

Weight Gain

The general consensus is that pregnant women of normal weight should gain 25-35lb. If they are overweight to start, they should only gain 15-25lb. Women who were underweight to start should gain 28-40lb. The recommendations are around 4lb in the first trimester, then a pound a week after that. We do NOT need to eat for two! This is totally a myth. During the 3rd trimester, you'll need an extra 450 calories per day.

A lot of women worry that increased insulin needs will lead to excessive weight gain. Just remember, non-diabetic mamas also make increased insulin to compensate for the insulin resistance caused by the placental hormones. Take what you need, but there's no need to take extra insulin simply for the sake of eating lots of carbohydrates.

Pumping in the 3rd Trimester

Q: I'm 29 weeks and have a lot of insulin resistance. My insulin pump doesn't seem to keep up with the larger boluses and I've had a few pods leak out insulin while delivering a mealtime bolus. I'm also having to change my reservoir frequently because I'm using so much insulin. What should I do?

A: At this point in pregnancy, you are likely taking a LOT of insulin and boluses can be quite large, especially if you aren't eating low carb (even if you are). I got down to a 1:2 insulin to carb ratio with my low carb baby so even low carb, that's a lot of insulin! Many find that they run out of insulin before 3 days are up and others experience issues like yours in addition to frequent pump failures and occlusions due to lack of good pump sites. You may find that it's helpful to pump for basal and to inject for boluses (or vice-versa). It will extend the life of your pump and you'll get better delivery. If you've read Dr. B's book, you'll remember that he says not to inject more than 7 units in one place (absorption becomes less reliable after 7 units) so it's a good idea to inject large doses in multiple sites. You'll almost definitely get better results than your pump boluses by doing this.

Pregnancy-Induced Hypertension

Pregnancy induced hypertension (PIH) is high blood pressure during pregnancy. It is defined as a systolic blood pressure (the upper number) higher than 140mmHg and a diastolic pressure (the lower number) higher than 90mmHg. PIH has 4 categories: a. preexisting hypertension (high blood pressure that you already had prior to pregnancy), b. gestational (only during pregnancy) hypertension, c. preexisting hypertension PLUS gestational hypertension and d. unclassifiable hypertension.

PIH can cause major problems and put mom and baby at high risk for multiple complications including prematurity and stillbirth. Women who have diabetes or preexisting hypertension are typically started on antihypertensive medications such as Methyldopa, Nifedipine or Labetalol once blood pressure rises above 140/90mm/hG. You may be placed on bed-rest, or hospitalized if blood pressure levels become too high.

Preeclampsia

As previously mentioned, type 1's are at increased risk for preeclampsia. While swollen feet can be normal (though miserable) swollen hands and face are NOT. If you experience this, or a severe headache, blurred vision, or high blood pressure, call your doctor immediately. They will test your urine for protein and run blood work. While the only cure for preeclampsia is delivery, it can be treated with Magnesium Sulfate and bedrest. If early delivery is necessary, baby has a much higher chance of survival at this point (though of course we want baby to stay in as long as possible).

Hemolysis, Elevated Liver, Low Platelets (HELLP) Syndrome

This is a condition in pregnancy that is associated with preeclampsia. If you develop HELLP syndrome, it is an emergency and needs urgent treatment. HELLP syndrome is a condition of the liver and blood. It stands for:

Hemolysis - the breakdown of red blood cells in your body. Red blood cells carry oxygen, so are very important.

Elevated Liver enzymes - an indication that there is a problem with your liver.

Low Platelets-platelets help your blood clot.

Symptoms of HELLP syndrome include fatigue or lethargy, pain in the upper abdomen, nausea, vomiting, headache, as well as swelling, sudden weight gain, blurry vision, shoulder pain and pain with breathing. Call your doctor right away if you experience these symptoms. If you develop HELLP syndrome late in your pregnancy, delivery of the baby should solve the problem. If you're earlier in the pregnancy, you may need blood transfusions, magnesium sulfate infusion, blood pressure medication and steroids to help your baby's lungs develop faster.

Pruritic Urticarial Papules and Plaques of Pregnancy (PUPPP)

PUPPP is an itchy rash some pregnant women get on their abdomen. It's most commonly found in first-time mamas, and in women who are carrying multiples. The rash can appear as pink- or skin-colored bumps. PUPPP is uncomfortable but is not dangerous. You can try things like a cold compress or an oatmeal bath to relieve the itching. If the itching becomes unbearable, contact your physician.

Intrahepatic Cholestasis

This is a condition that can happen, usually in late pregnancy. The main symptom is severe itching. Most mamas experience some mild itching due to your belly stretching, or PUPPP, but if he itching is disrupting your daily life, it might be something more. Intrahepatic cholestasis of pregnancy is a disorder in which the bile builds up in the liver due to a problem with bile release in the liver. There can also be yellowing of the skin and whites of the eyes (jaundice). This condition is associated with premature delivery and stillbirth, so if you experience severe itching, let your doctor know right away. The bile release goes back to normal after delivery of the baby typically.

Bladder Pressure

Q: I feel like I constantly have to pee! I'm not talking about every so often I need to go. I mean I'm sitting on the toilet and still have the sensation of needing to go badly. It's driving me nuts! Is this normal?

A: As you progress in your 3rd trimester, your baby is getting bigger and is likely head down, which puts pressure on your bladder. This can create the sensation that you have to pee all the time. The level you are talking about sounds like it could be a urinary tract infection (UTI) however. Your doctor can run a urinalysis to make sure you don't, and if you do, will put you on an antibiotic to clear it up. A UTI (urinary tract infection) can cause contractions and possibly preterm labor. Make sure you're drinking plenty of water, wiping front to back and urinating right after sex. All these things can help prevent a UTI.

Pelvic Pain

Q: I'm 31 weeks and completely miserable. It hurts when I move my legs. Getting out of a car is excruciating and it's even hard to roll over in bed! If I sit on the floor, my hubby has to pull me up. I'm having so much pelvic pain it feels like the bone in my crotch was kicked with a steel toed boot and broken! It's hard for me to walk and even getting dressed is nearly impossible. It's almost unbearable. My MFM and OB keep saying everything is fine and that it's just pregnancy. Is there anything that can help me? I don't know how much more I can take.

A: This sounds like Symphysis Pubis Dysfunction. It happens when the muscles and ligaments in your pelvis relax, due to a hormone called relaxin, which is preparing your body for labor. The pelvic joints become stiff and uneven. You may even hear a clicking noise when you move!

Approximately 1 in 35 women experience severe pain due to SPD. In the most severe state, known as diastasis of the symphysis pubis, when the joints completely separate.

This can cause excruciating pain and can cause problems during labor, necessitating cesarean section.

There is hope however! Find a chiropractor who is certified in the Webster technique. Chiropractic intervention can be exceedingly beneficial. Other tips include a pregnancy support belt, using a pillow between your legs when sleeping, taking tiny steps, avoiding lifting, and twisting, bending at the knees, avoiding the straddling position, and avoiding crossing your legs.

Chapter 13: Weeks 33-36

In the Home Stretch

You are so close! At this point, you're probably miserable, and can't wait to be done. I was always heavily pregnant in the summer, so it was especially miserable. You're probably thinking about the oncoming birth and getting ready for the baby. This is such an exciting time!

This is the time to start thinking about (if you haven't already) what your expectations are during labor. Will you keep your pump on? Will you have a glucose and insulin drip? What about your diet in the hospital? What to pack? How will your blood sugars be managed? What if you have a c-section? What if the baby's blood sugar is low? So many things to think about, and this is the time to discuss them with your doctor! Much of this chapter will be covering things to discuss with your doctor about your upcoming birth.

The Pump: to Keep or Not?

This is a personal choice between you and your doctor. I personally wanted to keep my pump during delivery.

During my first c-section, I kept my pump, and everything went perfectly. Blood sugars were beautiful, and baby did not have low blood sugar. With number 2, my MFM took my pump, but didn't put me on an insulin drip (afraid of hypos) and I spiked. Baby was born with low blood sugar which was very stressful. By the time baby number three came along, I made sure my doctor approved of my keeping my pump on, and numbers were perfect. No hypoglycemia for Adrian.

Many doctors prefer to keep their patients on a glucose and insulin drip so they can tightly manage numbers and for some mamas, this is a relief, not to have to deal with their diabetes. I always compromised and had a Dextrose I.V. available in case I dropped. It was never needed.

Hospital Food

Hospital food is notoriously bad, but not only is it bad tasting, it's horrible on blood sugars. They feed you a lot of starch and fruit, keeping things low-fat and low salt, while using a sliding scale for blood sugars which results in a nasty roller-coaster ride.

Excerpt from Allison's Pregnancy Blog

(Author's Note: this was during my hospitalization for mild DKA)

> *Dietary calls to take my dinner order but since there is no menu in my room, I must get the regular dinner which consists of Salisbury steak, russet potatoes, cornbread, and pound cake! I protested that I am a diabetic, but the lady stated that these foods were allowed for diabetics and didn't give me an option to change.*
>
> *The nurse came in later and asked about my dinner. She brought me a menu and told me to call and change my order. I am told that it is too late, and I cannot change my order. I again bring up the fact that my blood sugar is over 300 and I don't need to be eating all those carbs. The lady starts getting nasty and yells "they are allowed foods, there are no sugars in them!". No sugar in cornbread or pound cake? Ok. At this point the nurse takes the phone and states that I will not be eating that food and to please change my order. So, I finally got a nice dinner of beef stir fry with broccoli and my blood sugars slowly came down.*

I was very worried about food in the hospital and was concerned that I would not be allowed to eat during labor (many hospitals only allow ice chips). Well let me tell you, I had NO interest in eating anything. I couldn't focus on anything but my contractions. Food was the last thing on my mind.

Find out if your hospital allows you to order from a menu or if everyone receives the same thing. Ask your doctor to order you a REGULAR diet, not a diabetic diet. This will allow you to order low carb items and not be restricted on fat and sodium. If you don't have the choice to order, ask your significant other/birth partner to bring you in food.

Blood Glucose Management

Not only is the food in the hospital bad, but diabetes management is unfortunately abysmal for the most part. Most L&D nurses have not dealt with T1's or have very little experience. Blood sugar is checked at most, every four hours and a sliding scale is used to correct high blood sugars. No carb counting, no correction factor. It's completely reactive. It's all about correcting highs and preventing lows rather than avoiding highs in the first place!

Talk to your doctor about glucose management in the hospital. Request to check your own blood sugars with your meter or cgm and to have full control of your diabetes management. I just let the nurses know what my blood sugar was, and how much insulin I took. Do NOT allow your insulin and supplies to be confiscated. This leaves you powerless and in danger of DKA if some uninformed nurse decides to hold your basal (it happens all the time).

I.V. Fluids

You'll almost definitely have an I.V. when you have your baby. You will at least have a saline lock (where the cannula is inserted in your vein and taped down with no fluids going just in case you need to have a c-section, or to receive antibiotics or blood if needed). Make sure that your I.V. fluids are not giving you a caloric substance such as Dextrose (D5) or Lactate (LR) both of which will increase blood sugar levels. According to Dr. Bernstein, Normal Saline or Half Normal Saline are perfectly adequate for routine hydration. A dextrose I.V. the bag can be hanging, but only connected in case of lows. Discuss this with your doctor beforehand and have it noted in your orders, normal saline, or half normal saline only.

If you're wondering about why Lactated Ringers is off the table as it isn't dextrose, that comes down to the Cori Cycle. Lactate is converted to pyruvate which is converted to glucose.

Will I be Induced?

The biggest question for me was whether to induce. At the beginning of the pregnancy, I was hell-bent on waiting until he came naturally, or at least going to 40 weeks.

Throughout the pregnancy, I developed some moderate (and at times severe) anxiety about the worst possible outcomes. I think this must be common for Type 1 women since we have grown up hearing about complications and fetal death. As the pregnancy went on, and we met so many milestones, and my love for my little boy intensified beyond what I knew was possible, my mindset changed.

Even though my control was so tight, and knowing that complications are related to poor control, I started considering induction at 39 weeks. I had read the Arrive studies and know so many kids that were born early - all of whom are thriving. By the end of the pregnancy, I was comfortable being induced at 39 weeks, and my OB wanted this as well (though she was very nervous about going beyond 38 weeks since the MFM had recommended no later than 38 weeks).

At 38 weeks and 2 days, I suddenly had severe hypoglycemia and my insulin needs plummeted by at least 50%. Knowing this was a sign of placental failure, I was terrified something was wrong and went to the hospital.

Everything was fine - placenta was fine - baby was great. However, the experience was frightening, and I agreed to be induced two days later. Looking back, this was the right decision for me, and even though it was fear induced, I don't regret it at all.

I had a great labor and delivered at 38 weeks and 5 days. I went into the hospital prepared to go to war with anyone who fought me on my insulin regimen. But I never had to use any of my letters or research articles - the nurses and staff were completely understanding. In fact, they were incredibly interested in my level of control and how I did it. Throughout the day, and the next day, I had a handful of medical staff come and talk to me about my diabetes and how I was able to be so controlled and have such a healthy baby. I was so thrilled to share my story!

After a few hours of labor (with an epidural) and 30 minutes of pushing (yes - I was very lucky), I popped out the most perfect little 6-pound 1 ounce, 19.5-inch baby boy. Our little Rockstar is as healthy as could be!"

-Olivia

If you are type 1, there is a high likelihood that your doctor will want to induce labor. Early induction is one of my huge pet-peeves. A large majority of doctors routinely induce labor between 37 and 38 weeks for type 1's regardless of control. According to **ACOG** (the American College of Obstetrics and Gynecology), "The College and SMFM have long recommended that doctors do not induce labor or perform cesareans before 39 weeks of pregnancy without a clear medical reason. A full-term pregnancy lasts 40 weeks. "Early-term" deliveries are those that occur between 37 and 39 weeks of gestation.

"There are certain medical indications that require early delivery, including preeclampsia/eclampsia, fetal growth restriction, placental abruption, multiple fetuses, and POORLY CONTROLLED DIABETES. However, suspecting that a baby is macrosomic (large) is not an indication to induce or deliver by cesarean before 39 weeks."

ACOG recommends that well-controlled pregestational diabetics be delivered between 39 0/7 weeks and 39 6/7 weeks. If blood sugars are not well-controlled, or if you have vascular complications, it is recommended to deliver between 36 0/7 weeks and 38 6/7 weeks. (ACOG 2019)

Diabetes alone is not an indication for early delivery! Suspected macrosomia (big baby) is also not an indication for early delivery according to ACOG. It is also not an indication for cesarean unless the baby is estimated to be greater than 4500g (remember those ultrasounds can be very wrong though!) If my doctor told me I will be having a cesarean based only on diabetes, I would RUN. Ask these questions early on so you can find a supportive provider.

Timing of delivery — We and others see little benefit in continuing pregnancy beyond 39 weeks in women with diabetes and thus suggest induction of labor for these pregnancies by 40 weeks of gestation. Preterm delivery should be avoided, except when glycemic control is suboptimal or there are other maternal or fetal reasons for concern (e.g., maternal vascular disease). In these cases, an acceptable approach is to induce labor at 36+0 to 38+6 weeks (or earlier depending on the specific clinical setting). When such a plan is chosen, the risks of a prolonged induction due to an unfavorable cervix must be weighed against the risks associated with continuing the pregnancy.

- UpToDate

Additional studies and articles

Women with well-controlled diabetes, normal antenatal testing, and normally grown fetuses can go into spontaneous labor, with induction reserved until approximately 40 weeks' gestation. Early delivery without maternal or fetal indication in women with diabetes is no longer the norm unless fetal lung maturity is documented. Cesarean delivery should be reserved for other obstetric indications, fetal compromise, or estimated fetal weight greater than 4500 g.

- *http://www.ncbi.nlm.nih.gov/pmc/articles/PMC3385360/*

We believe that with a lack of solid evidence to justify routine intervention based on any type of threshold, the decision on elective delivery should be made on an individual basis, taking into account a number of clinical factors including gestational age, sonographic and clinical.

- https://www.ncbi.nlm.nih.gov/pmc/articles/PMC4934937/

Estimated fetal weight, type of diabetes, degree of glycemic control, obstetrical history of the individual patient (e.g., a history of stillbirth) as well as parity and cervical status. The potential benefits and risks of elective delivery should be discussed with the patient, and patient preference following such a discussion should also be included in the final decision on elective delivery.

-https://www.ncbi.nlm.nih.gov/pmc/articles/PMC4900972/

For women with well-controlled diabetes, whether pregestational or gestational, a late preterm or early term birth, i.e., before 39 completed weeks of gestation, is not indicated. In a setting of poorly controlled diabetes, an individualized decision aiming for late preterm or early term delivery (before 38 weeks + 6 days gestation) is recommended. An early term or term delivery (38–39 weeks + 6 days gestation) is suggested if vascular complications are present in women with pregestational diabetes.

-https://www.aafp.org/afp/2003/1101/p1767.html

"There are no indications to pursue delivery before 40 weeks of gestation in patients with good glycemic control unless other maternal or fetal indications are present."

The fact is, early induction while logical, is not evidence-based. It is standard protocol by most doctors, but there is no research backing it. This is a serious decision between you and your doctor. Do your research. Read the literature. Make your own decision based on what's best for you and your baby.

I would not agree to an induction unless there was an express clinical reason. I saw MWs for my last 3 pregnancies. With the 1st MW, we decided that we'd wait & evaluate based on BPP/NST at 38wks then play it by ear from there- baby was "BIG" and MFM wanted to induce at 38.5wk, I declined. MW was supportive- I went into labor the next day & easily birthed my 10lb boy (my first baby was no peanut 9lb3oz). Next 2 pregnancies were a different MW, similar plan- wait & see, BPP/NST only if we had any concerns or I went post-date. Baby 3 was born 40wks 9.5lbs, baby 4, 41wks 7.5lbs (born en route to the hospital, oops!)"

-Rachel Fontenault

What about the risk of stillbirth?

This is of course a very scary thought, and nobody wants to risk losing their baby, but we have to think about a couple things here. The risk of stillbirth is very low.

Waiting for labor to start on its own is reasonable if blood glucose levels are well-controlled and the mother and baby are doing well. However, extending pregnancy beyond 40 to 41 weeks of gestation is generally not recommended; some practitioners routinely induce labor between 39 and 40 weeks in all women with type 1 or 2 diabetes.

The risk of stillbirth for pregnant women with well-controlled diabetes is very low and is about the same as in women without diabetes (less than 1 percent). The mortality (death) rate in infants of diabetic women is slightly higher than in nondiabetics (2 versus 1 percent).

This is mostly due to a higher rate of serious birth defects in infants of diabetic mothers. Before insulin became available in 1922, women with diabetes mellitus were at very high risk of complications of pregnancy. Today, most women with diabetes can have a safe pregnancy and delivery, similar to that of nondiabetic women.

This was a reasonable approach prior to 1950 since one-half of stillbirths in this population occurred after the 38th week of gestation. However, fetal mortality has fallen precipitously among both diabetic women and the general obstetric population over the past few decades; thus, for most patients, the morbidity and mortality from prematurity and failed induction should be weighed carefully against contemporary estimates of potential benefit from early delivery.

The incidence of late fetal death in pregnancies complicated by diabetes mellitus, which was 50 percent in the pre-insulin era, has been steadily falling, presumably due to stricter glycemic control and improvements in obstetrical and neonatal care [42,43]. The stillbirth rate in women with optimal glycemic control now approaches that of nondiabetic women [43-45], especially in the absence of macrosomia and polyhydramnios. Congenital malformations now account for approximately 50 percent of the perinatal deaths in infants of diabetic mothers.

- UpToDate

Some doctors will argue that the risk is still inherent, no matter the level of control, but as previously stated earlier in the book, those risks are based on "tight control" of an a1c of less than 6.9%, nearly double normal blood sugar! Early induction for the prevention of stillbirth is logical, but it is not evidence-based. Studies are lacking when it comes to this. Early induction may decrease the likelihood of macrosomia, but evidence is lacking that it improves outcomes.

Other things to consider; if your body is not ready to deliver, i.e., your cervix is unfavorable, there is a high likelihood that you will end up with a cesarean. Induction on its own increases the likelihood of cesarean as medical induction causes intense contractions unlike what your body would experience in natural labor, and many women will need an epidural, which can slow down the progression of labor, resulting in a cesarean.

My first two babies were taken around 38 weeks and with my third, I went to 40 weeks (39 by their count, but I know when I conceived, so it worked out to my benefit!). My MFM had stated that I could go to 41 weeks because my control was so good, but they had scared me so much by telling me my baby would be macrosomic and likely more than 10lb (WRONG) that I decided to go early. Stillbirth does happen, and it is likely the most horrible thing that a mom can experience (other than losing a child in general). If blood sugars are not normal, please take every precaution. Don't take a risk. If your blood sugars *are* normal, do your research, discuss this with your doctor, and make the decision that is right for you.

Will I Need a Cesarean?

Diabetes alone is **NOT** an indication for cesarean, and if your doctors tell you you're going to have a cesarean based only on your being type 1, run fast! Suspected macrosomia is not an indication unless the baby is estimated to be larger than 4500g and as I've said repeatedly, ultrasound estimates can be very off!

Some *actual* indications for cesarean section might include placenta previa, severe pre-eclampsia (toxemia), a prior cesarean with a *classical* incision (not a low transverse incision which is most common), breech presentation*, failure to progress (though this is debatable because some doctors will call it failure to progress after a specific time limit, like 12 hours and sometimes it takes longer! I stayed at 4-5 for something like 14 hours, but my VBAC was still successful) multiple gestation, HIV, absolute disproportion (your pelvis is too small-this is VERY rare, and the doctor cannot tell this just by looking at you!), chorioamnionitis (amniotic infection), transverse presentation, to name a few.

*See "Breech Baby" section.

Sometimes a c-section absolutely *is* necessary and is lifesaving, but all too many times, it is done unnecessarily, especially to women with diabetes.

Author's Story: Aiden's Birth

Aidan Matthew Herschede arrived Nov 1, at 10:26 am via c-section. He was 8lb even and 20 in. long. I checked into the hospital the night before so I could get settled and they could monitor my blood sugars. They hooked me up to the monitors, started my IV etc.

The next morning about 9:30 they wheeled me to the operating room. They did have some trouble getting my spinal in which was not fun, but after it was in, everything was fine. They disconnected my pump, as I had grudgingly agreed to an insulin drip after the c-section until after I was eating solid foods.

The c-section went by very smoothly, and my little boy cried from the minute he came out nonstop! His first blood sugar was fine, but after that it started to drop, so they gave him some Nutramigen from a syringe (we are in the TRIGR study). I was in recovery for a couple hours and they still had not started my insulin drip, and I was getting

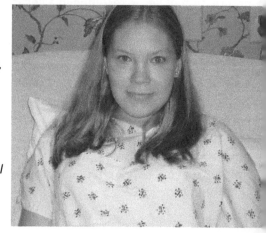

agitated. I kept asking, and they said that the doctor had ordered a sliding scale to correct, but did not order a drip. I let them give me two units for a 180 and then an hour later it had not come down and they wanted to give me 6 units of Regular subcutaneously, which really made me mad, and refused it at first, but finally gave in as I knew my blood sugar would not come down on its own. I demanded to talk to my doctor about it, and they said I could talk to him when he got out of c-sections.

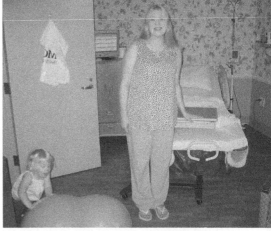

He finally came in and said he decided not to put me on the drip because he was afraid I that would drop down. GRRRR! My sugars stayed pretty stable, but by morning I was 200 and I got fed up and put my pump back on. My blood sugar was fine after this. Aidan took right to nursing, and had no problems latching on. I went home after three days, and we are doing fine. I am not bouncing back as quickly this time, and have had more pain than last time, but overall am doing well. My blood sugars have been perfect, except for some lows after nursing. He's a little bigger than I thought he'd be, but he is a healthy and happy baby!

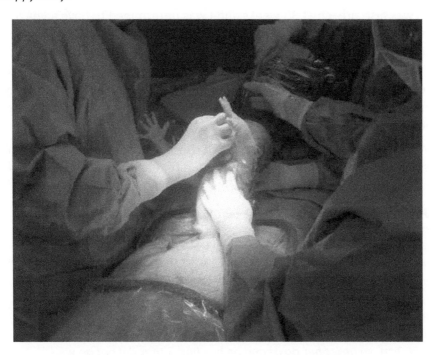

Breech Baby

My first pregnancy was delivered by a scheduled cesarean section because my daughter was breech (she was coming butt first rather than headfirst). The first inclination of most doctors is to perform a cesarean when your baby is breech. That said, a breech baby *CAN* be delivered vaginally, but the doctor or midwife needs to be experienced in this, and there is risk involved. There are other measures that can be taken too, such as an external cephalic version, or in layman's terms, the doctor physically turns the baby around using his hands (from the outside).

I tried everything I could think of to get Diana to turn, including jumping on a trampoline, standing on my head, and lying upside down on an inverted ironing board.

Nothing worked. Part of me feels like if she had been given more time (taken at 37w6d) she might have turned on her own. I was scheduled for an external version that day, and prior to this, I had an amniocentesis performed to check the baby's lung maturity. During this procedure, my MFM doctor had a hard time getting fluid because it was low (oligohydramnios). My AFI (amniotic fluid index) was a 6 and he said it would be too dangerous to turn her. I asked couldn't I drink lots of water to bring it up, and I was told this wouldn't work. Later, during my third pregnancy, my AFI was a 6 and I drank lots of water. Two days later I was at a 15!

Adrian was also breech at 35 weeks and I was determined to have a vba2c. I found the website, www.spinningbabies.com which was super helpful in learning the exact position the baby is lying (belly mapping) and methods to get him to turn. The method that worked turned out to be playing loud music between my legs. It did take a while, so be patient. I physically felt him turn around (very weird and uncomfortable sensation I must say) and from then he stayed head down.

The Webster Technique (mentioned previously in the question about Symphysis Pubis Dysfunction) is a chiropractic technique that has proven very successful in getting a breech baby to turn as well so is definitely worth considering.

VBAC: Vaginal Birth After C-Section

Excerpt from Allison's Pregnancy Blog

The Dr. said that he will allow me to VBAC if that's what I really want, but he wants me to think seriously about the pros and cons before I make a decision. The risk of uterine rupture is around 3% and while this is a low number, for those 3% it is devastating. * He said he has had HUNDREDS of successful VBACs including one recently after THREE cesareans (she came in at 9cm, so he let her do it) and he has had 3 that did not go well.

One infant did not make it, one is mentally handicapped and with the other, the baby is fine, but mom had to have a hysterectomy. Those are scary things to think about and I will have to think long and hard about it. He also said that he will not take the baby early unless absolutely necessary, and that he will let me go to 40 or 41 weeks!

Let's hope we can go before that.

(Author's Note) After additional research, it turns out the risk is actually lower than this. According to the American Pregnancy Association, the risk of uterine rupture after 2 previous cesareans is less than 1%.

This is a topic which is very near and dear to my heart. When I was a young child, my family was a member of a church where home birth was very common. At baby showers, women would watch videos of other mamas' home births or birthing center births. My mom also had a copy of *A Child is Born*, a book about pregnancy and childbirth which has some pretty graphic pictures of childbirth. I was exposed to natural birth from a very young age and always imagined myself giving birth this way. Alas, homebirth was not something that would be a part of my future, nor a midwife assisted birthing center birth. My cesareans were traumatic. During my first, the spinal anesthesia had not been administered correctly (apparently, I was not given enough medication) and I started feeling the c-section halfway through. I remember laying there on the table and the doctor is talking about being up in his deer stand and I am yelling, "hey, I feel that!" "That hurts!" Finally, he paid attention to my cries and put me under. Afterward they let Matt take the baby around to see the family, then they kept her in observation for 6 hours due to 'protocol'. It was hell. I was crying and begging to see my baby.

The only reason Diana was kept in observation was my diabetes, which I think is ridiculous. Her temperature and blood sugar could have been monitored right there in the room with me. By the time #2 came around, I knew I didn't want another cesarean and asked my MFM about VBAC. He nodded that it was certainly a possibility and I likely could have a VBAC. As the time drew nearer to my delivery, he changed his tune, however. "I can by looking at you that you cannot deliver vaginally".

I remember them bringing the consent papers in.

Nurse: "You are agreeing to an elective repeat cesarean section".

Me: "No, this isn't elective, he's making me have a c-section".

Silence.

Nurse: "Your alternative is a vaginal delivery".

Me: "No, he won't let me have a vaginal delivery."

Again, silence. I looked around the room at the birthing ball, the birthing bar, the birthing tub, and broke down sobbing. The nurse looked at me like I was stupid.

The spinal anesthesia was painful, and I stressed the importance of them giving me enough medication as I had experienced a lot of pain with my previous Cesarean. I was given so much that I was numb up to my chest and kept forgetting to breathe.

Afterward, they wouldn't let me see my baby as there were no infant CPR certified nurses in recovery. I laid there crying for my baby as my blood sugar crept up.

My doctor had not put me on an insulin drip for fear of hypos, (despite forcing me to remove my insulin pump) and my blood sugar was 180mg/dL. They told me I could talk to him when he was done doing c-sections. The next morning, I was up to 200mg/dL. I put my pump back on without permission and everything was fine after that.

I went home very sore and had immense pain which continued for 6 weeks. I couldn't even stand because I was in so much pain. The Army hospital ruled out appendicitis and gave me Tylenol and Motrin, which did nothing. I was in so much agony, at my 6 weeks checkup, I begged the doctor to do something.

He did an ultrasound and said my body was reacting to an internal stitch and was fighting it off like a foreign invader, thus the swelling and pain. He gave me Percocet, which allowed me to function while I single-handedly cleaned and packed up our apartment to move to Fort Stewart, GA, where Matt had been stationed and had already been sent. All while taking care of an infant and a two-year old.

Aidan's birth traumatized me, and I mourned my lost births. I tell people I was depressed for 5 years afterward.

When I got pregnant with #3, I was determined to have a vba2c (vaginal birth after 2 cesareans). I spent hours upon hours reading about VBA2C and finding a VBAC friendly provider. I found out ACOG's new policies. ACOG had recently put out the following statement, "Attempting a vaginal birth after cesarean (VBAC) is a safe and appropriate choice for most women who have had a prior cesarean delivery, including for some women who have had two previous cesareans, according to guidelines released today by The American College of Obstetricians and Gynecologists."

What is the risk of VBAC? The main risk is uterine rupture which is not something to take lightly. It is something that is very serious and could result in having to have a hysterectomy, losing your baby, or bleeding out. If rapid action is taken when a rupture happens, mom and baby typically do well. The risk is very low, however. For women who have had one cesarean section with a horizontal incision (low transverse) the risk of uterine rupture is 0.72%. The risk is lowered if the first cesarean was closed with double-layer sutures. I obtained a copy of my operative report and they actually used THREE layers of sutures. Pregnancy should be at least 18-24 months after the previous pregnancy. Misoprostol (Cytotek) should be completely avoided for induction.

I also concluded that inducing at 38 weeks was outdated and unnecessary if I kept tight control. I was eating low carb this time around which made things much smoother with much fewer hypos than my previous pregnancies.

Steve Cooksey worked with me for numerous hours getting through that pregnancy. I am forever grateful.

I found a wonderful MFM doctor who also had a midwife who followed me. He agreed that I could go to 40 or 41 weeks if things were going well and that if I wanted to attempt a VBA2C. He also agreed to let me keep my pump and CGMS on and ordered a normal diet for me so I could pick what I wanted and eat low carb.

Adrian Christopher was born via induced vba2c after 20 hours of labor. No complications. No NICU time. No neonatal hypoglycemia. He was not 10+lb as they had predicted, but 8lb12oz and 21.5 inches long, so he was big everywhere and not macrosomic.

I had a successful vba2c at 40 weeks gestation. Practically unheard of for a type 1 diabetic. The biggest piece of advice that I can give for successful advice is to find a VBAC friendly provider. If the doctor says, "you may be able to have a VBAC *if* you go into labor by 38 weeks, *if* the baby isn't too big, *if* your labor doesn't last more than 12 hours", with a whole list of *if's*, they are likely not truly supportive of VBAC.

Questions to ask; if you are allowed a TOLAC (trial of labor after cesarean) will you be allowed to labor in a regular room or be required to labor in the operating room? My birthing room was right next door to the operating room so they could rush me in if necessary. What kind of monitoring does your doctor require? Will you be allowed to get up and move around? I was required to be on the fetal monitor the entire time and wasn't even allowed to get up to use the bathroom! I had been told prior that the hospital had wireless monitors, but when I got there, they told me they didn't! Find out for sure. Will your doctor induce if you don't go into labor in time? I was induced with a Foley Bulb (they insert a urinary catheter into your cervix and inflate the little balloon which manually dilates your cervix) which ended up being successful with a tiny bit of Pitocin when I stalled. Some doctors will not induce a VBAC. Find out all these things when selecting a doctor. **ICAN** (International Cesarean Awareness Network) is very helpful, and your local chapter should be able to help you find a VBAC friendly provider. You can also google "VBAC friendly providers" in your area.

A member of one of my long-time pregnancy groups had this advice for a successful VBAC:

> *How I beat the odds to have a successful T1D VBAC:*
>
> 1. *Researched hospital stats to learn which of the six hospitals in my area had the highest statistics of VBAC success. One hospital was clearly superior to the others in this regard, with 18% of all births occurring there being VBAC, and an 85% VBAC success rate. (This hospital actually has the highest VBAC stats in the entire state.)*
>
> 2. *Hired the most liberal Perinatologist in the region -- who happens to also work at the previously determined VBAC-friendly hospital of choice. (For example, he is known as being the only doctor in this region willing to attend vaginal births of breech babies.)*
>
> 3. *Fortunately, my current Endo also works at this same VBAC-friendly hospital.*
>
> 4. *Hired Integrated Diabetes Services* to help me manage my blood sugars throughout pregnancy. (The CDE at my Endo's doesn't do pregnant T1Ds very often.) My CDE at the coaching service helps pregnant T1Ds all the time; for example, she had 4 clients give birth within 2 weeks of me.*
>
> 5. *Hired a doula who specializes in supporting moms attempting a VBAC.*
>
> 6. *Went to a chiropractor regularly throughout the pregnancy.*
>
> 7. *Aimed to eat 80 grams of protein per day.*
>
> 8. *Took a great childbirth education course (Hypnobabies).*
>
> 9. *Politely declined almost all 3rd trimester testing, including weekly amniotic fluid level checks, twice a week non-stress tests (I only did it once a week), and all growth scans.*
>
> 10. *Labored at home until pushing began, arriving at the hospital ready to deliver. (Afterwards, my doctor said, "That's the way to do it! Show up without giving anyone at the hospital time to interfere!")*
>
> *If any of you are wanting to VBAC, I encourage you to go for it!*
>
> -Elizabeth

*Integrated Diabetes Services is a diabetes and pregnancy coaching service. I have heard nothing but good things about them. I also offer diabetes and pregnancy coaching through **diaVerge Diabetes**. You can find more info at diaverge.com.

On Maxwell

In 2019, I became pregnant with my son. At this point, I had been eating low carb for over four years and felt very confident in my abilities to manage my blood sugar well throughout pregnancy. To be honest, I was thrown for a loop early on in the first trimester. I experienced respiratory illness and had a lot of travel and stress, which, unfortunately, contributed to less than desirable blood glucose levels on some occasions. It seemed that I was much more insulin resistant in the first trimester than during the pregnancy with my daughter, which was frustrating, but manageable, once I accepted that this was a new experience, and I just had to make the adjustments needed in terms of insulin dosing. Although I was disappointed with my management early on (my A1c in the first trimester was 5.8%), I was able to achieve A1c levels of <5.4% for the remainder of the pregnancy.

This time around, I worked with a regular OB. They were comfortable with caring for me and really treated me as an individual. I felt they listened to me and I much preferred them to my MFM team.

My endocrinologist was a forward-thinking APRN, whom I saw just twice during the pregnancy. He even joked with me about how he was writing my insulin prescriptions based on the assumption that I was eating 50 g of carbohydrates per meal. I still remember that conversation. He said, "I know you're not doing that! Because you'd never have numbers like this, if you were."

I managed all of my insulin adjustments. It was nice to have my Endo's support in terms of agreeing that I knew exactly what I was doing, and even more so, when it came time to write a letter of support to circumvent the hospital protocols of insulin management during delivery. Everyone worked together to make the delivery experience a smooth one, and I am grateful that I found a team of thoughtful and caring providers.

The pregnancy was largely uneventful, overall. I attended the appointments and time and time again, everything was normal. One anecdote stands out. At 39 weeks pregnant I contracted a GI virus. I wasn't feeling so great and was almost resigned to having the baby by C-section because I did not think I could muster the energy to be in active labor. Thankfully, I got over it quickly. Believe it or not, based entirely on my intuition, the next morning I lowered my basal insulin from 25 U to 19 U, for the remainder of the pregnancy. I don't know why I chose this particular reduction, but it worked perfectly. A mother (or a long-standing type 1) just knows, I guess, to trust themselves to make choices they cannot always explain.

At 39 weeks and 3 days, I opted for a membrane sweep. I went into labor at 39 weeks and 4 days, just like with my daughter. I labored without pain medication for over 12 hours. My labor stalled and Pitocin was started. I used nitrous oxide gas to help manage the pain for several hours, but I was still not making much progress. Finally, I opted for an epidural and to have my water broken. About 6 hours later, I delivered my son via spontaneous VBAC.

He was born weighing 7 lb. 11 oz. He inhaled a bit of fluid on his way out, but he did well soon after that and was able to stay in the room with us. He scored well on the APGARs and did not experience hypoglycemia. He had a slight touch of jaundice, but we were able to be discharged about 36 hours after birth.

I was thrilled to manage my own blood glucose levels throughout labor and delivery, too. Everything went smoothly and I was able to balance the experience with monitoring my blood sugar and making the appropriate adjustments.

My recovery was fantastic, and we are still breastfeeding, 11 months later.

-Maria Muccioli, PhD, Diabetes Daily

With my second baby, I was eating low carb and got pregnant the very next month after we started trying. I was desperate to not have a c-section again, so I went to a bigger hospital and OB group with multiple OB's, most of whom were wonderful and very open to VBAC. They left my diabetes to me and my endo, which I appreciated, and I just showed them my blood sugar chart, but they didn't try to mess with it. My A1c's were only slightly better than before (5.8-6.1) but they thought I was doing a good job. My baby was head up about 32 weeks and they wanted to schedule a c-section, but I found some spinning babies exercises and he flipped by the next appointment. They consented to let me go to 40 weeks, but I actually went into labor at 38w6d and went to the hospital. I hadn't gotten any sleep the previous night from early labor and I was exhausted and in pain, especially since they wanted me on my back and on monitors, so I asked for an epidural. As soon as I was out of pain, I went to sleep and slept for 8 hours! I only tested my blood sugars a handful of times through the whole labor, without a CGM, and I had taken half my normal long-acting insulin.

When I woke up, I could not feel a thing in my lower half. The epidural was very strong for me, so I asked them to check my progression, and they said I was complete! 10 cm! They had to direct me when to push since I could not feel a thing and one of my legs was completely numb and paralyzed, so I had help to push that leg back. I pushed for about half an hour, but it seems short to me. He came out at 6lb5oz, which I attribute to my low carb diet, and again had slightly low blood sugar but not concerning and

*never needed sugar water. Labor was a total of 37 hours. I had a 2nd
degree tear, which was as painful healing as the c-section, but I was glad
to have had him what I considered to be the more healthy, natural way. He
breastfed great without any problems.*

-Katherine Witherell

Monitoring

At this point in your pregnancy, you'll likely be having weekly Non-Stress Tests
(NST's) and Biophysical Profiles (BPP's). Weight estimates are generally at least
once a month if you don't decline them.

Group B Strep

Around 35 weeks, most doctors will perform a swab for Group-B strep. This is
a bacterium that is normal vaginal flora for some women, but can be harmful
to the baby, so if you are positive, you'll be given antibiotics before a vaginal
delivery. It is a simple swab of the vaginal and rectal area and is not painful.
I was positive with my last two pregnancies. I was given Ampicillin in my I.V.
when they started my induction.

Leaking?

Q. I just felt a little gush of fluid and my underwear is wet. I'm not sure if I
peed myself or if I'm leaking amniotic fluid. What should I do?

A. Sometimes it can be hard to tell, as you have a lot of pressure on your
bladder, and you may be leaking urine. You can put on a pad and see if it
becomes wet. Amniotic fluid will be clear (not yellow like urine) and will
typically have no odor (urine definitely has an odor). Some mamas say that
the amniotic fluid smells slightly sweet. If you do think you are leaking
amniotic fluid, give your doctor a call as they can check and find out. The
tests the doctor does can actually be done at home if you have the proper
tools on hand.

- pH Paper - The normal pH of vaginal fluid
  is between 4.5-6. Amniotic fluid has a pH
  of 7.1-7.3. pH paper can be purchased
  from Amazon.

- Nitrazine Paper - These strips, which can
  also be purchased online measure the
  pH as well. They turn blue if pH is greater
  than 6. It can show a false positive if you
  have an infection, or if there is semen
  present in your vaginal fluid.

- Ferning Microscope - Testing your saliva for ferning is a method for detecting ovulation while trying to conceive. Due to high estrogen levels at the time of ovulation, saliva will show a ferning pattern. Amniotic fluid also shows a ferning pattern and if you happen to have a microscope from your ttc days, you could test it out.

All these items would need to be something you already have on hand. Don't wait if you think you are leaking. Call your doctor and get checked.

Decreased Movement

After feeling your baby move for a while, you start to know your baby's normal movement. If your baby isn't moving or is moving less than normal, don't just assume the baby is sleepy or "running out of room". Don't take a risk. Call your doctor and get checked. It is *always* better to be safe in these situations.

Contraction Timer

A contraction Timer is an app you can download to your mobile device to measure the duration (how low long it lasts) and frequency (how often it's happening) of your contractions. It can also help you measure the intensity (how strong they are). The app can help you determine your stage of labor, and whether it's time to call your doctor yet.

Chapter 14: Decreasing Insulin Needs

A Whole Chapter?

Yes! This topic is so important to me, I am dedicating a whole chapter to it.

This topic is o important to me. I see it multiple times a week in the pregnancy and diabetes groups. In the last sixteen years, I have observed this phenomenon in *NUMEROUS* T1 mamas; almost all of them I dare say. Usually somewhere between 34-36 weeks, there is a precipitous drop in insulin needs. You'll start running low all the time. When the woman tells her doctor about what's happening, he becomes very alarmed and states the placenta is failing and the baby must be born *NOW* or even perform an 'emergency' cesarean because the placenta is failing, and this is a dire situation!

I cannot *tell* you how many times I have watched this happen and it *KILLS* me.

I'll preface by saying, it is possible. A fall in insulin needs

can indicate that the placenta is failing, but it is typically not the case, and your doctor can check to find out. The blood flow to and from the placenta can be checked via doppler. The placenta can be checked for calcifications via ultrasound. The level of the hormone, Human Placental Lactogen can be checked from a sample of your blood. The baby can be monitored via NST and BPP. All these things can tell you if your placenta is healthy or not. There is no reason to jump to an unnecessary induction or cesarean only based on falling insulin needs.

I was lucky enough that my MFM doctors all knew that this was normal and were not concerned at all. They did check the placenta and monitored the baby to give me peace of mind, and all was fine. This happened with all three of my babies at 35 weeks each time.

Study 1:

RESULTS:

We included 350 women (146 type 1, 204 type 2), of which 15% had a drop of ≥15% in third-trimester basal insulin requirements. There was no difference in the primary outcome between groups (aOR 0.75 [0.27, 1.81]). In isolation the sensitivity and specificity of a ≥15% drop in basal IR as a diagnostic test for the primary outcome was 13% and 85%, respectively.

CONCLUSION:

A ≥15% drop in third-trimester basal IR is not associated with and is a poor predictor of adverse pregnancy outcomes in women with pre-pregnancy diabetes. It should not be used in isolation as a sole indication for delivery.

Falling Insulin Requirements and Adverse Pregnancy Outcomes in Women with Pre-pregnancy Diabetes (Vainder, Marina MD; Natt, Navneet MD; D'Souza, Rohan D. MD, PhD; Syeda, Ambreen MD; Mitsakakis, Nicholas, Obstetrics & Gynecology: May 2020 - Volume 135 - Issue - p 41S)

Study 2:

RESULTS:

Our cohort consisted of 157 women: 30 Type 1, 43 Type 2 and 84 gestational diabetics. Twenty-one (13%) experienced a drop in insulin with an average decline of 28% starting at 34 weeks. There was no significant difference in complications related to placental dysfunction (33% vs 244%; P=.37). There was a significantly increased rate of polyhydramnios (43% vs 9%; P<.01).

Women who experienced a decline in insulin delivered one week earlier (median 36w44d vs. 37w44d; P<.01). NICU admissions rates were higher (62% vs. 33%; P<.01) independent of gestational age, and were secondary to respiratory distress (52% vs. 24%; P<.01) as there were no differences in rates of treated hypoglycemia.

CONCLUSION:

We found no relationship between a decline in insulin requirement and placental function related complications. Interestingly, we found higher rates of polyhydramnios and NICU admissions for respiratory distress regardless of gestational age, suggesting a decline in insulin requirement has a greater impact on the neonate after delivery.

(Declining Insulin Requirements in Late Pregnancy: A Cause for Concern? [07D] Wilkinson, Barbara E. MD, MA; McDonnell, Marie MD; Palermo, Nadine DO; Lassey, Sarah C. MD; Little, Sarah E. MD, MPH. Obstetrics & Gynecology: May 2020 - Volume 135 - Issue - p 40S

I personally have to wonder if the delivery one week earlier was due to the OBGYN inducing early due to a decline in insulin requirements. We know that respiratory distress is a complication of diabetes and pregnancy and therefore in *my* opinion, the baby should be delivered *later* to give the lungs more time to develop. Just my opinion.

I'm not a doctor.

Study 3:

RESULTS:

We identified 1011 publications, of which three observational studies met eligibility criteria. Two studies that used ≥15 PFID were included in the quantitative analysis. Pregnancies with ≥15 PFID were associated with small-for-gestational-age (SGA) fetuses (6/40 vs. 7/153, p=0.04; risk ratio (RR) 2.95 [1.08, 8.07]). There were no differences in large-for- gestational-age fetuses (14/40 vs. 58/153; RR 1.07 [0.68, 1.70]), low 5-minute Apgar scores (6/40 vs. 16/153; RR 1.93 [0.52, 7.14]), caesarean deliveries (25/40 vs. 105/153; RR 0.90 [0.70, 1.17]), extreme preterm (3/35 vs. 2/104) birth, stillbirths (1/35 vs. 1/104) or hypertensive disorders (9/35 vs. 19/104, p=0.34).

CONCLUSION:

This systematic review of observational studies found no association between ≥15 PFID and adverse pregnancy outcomes, except for a higher number of SGA fetuses. This was not causal. Early delivery based on ≥15 PFID cannot be recommended. Instead, clinical management should involve continued maternal-fetal surveillance, exploring possible obstetric and metabolic reasons for this PFID, and treatment of the primary cause.

Falling Third-Trimester Insulin Requirements and Adverse Pregnancy Outcomes: A Systematic Review [32E] Sayyar, Parastoo; Alavifard, Sepand BSc; D'Souza, Rohan MD, MSc, MRCO. Obstetrics & Gynecology: May 2018 - Volume 131 - Issue - p 61S

Study 4:

Implications of a fall in insulin requirements - Insulin requirements sometimes fail after 35 weeks of gestation. This is observed more often in women with type 1 diabetes than in women with gestational diabetes mellitus (GDM) and in women with longer durations of type 1 diabetes.

A fall in insulin dose greater than 5 to 10 percent should prompt assessment of fetal well-being and a search for medical conditions or other factors that could account for the drop. Decreasing insulin requirements are weakly associated with placental insufficiency as well as decreased

maternal intake or vomiting. If fetal well-being is confirmed, then a fall in insulin requirement is not associated with adverse fetal outcome and is not an indication for delivery. Decreased insulin requirements of up to 30 percent with good pregnancy outcome have been reported. The reduced need for insulin may be related to increased fetal demand for maternal glucose, increased maternal sensitivity to insulin in the fasting state, and/ or a decrease in human chorionic somatomammotropin (formerly human placental lactogen), which has been observed in women with GDM.

– UpToDate

A smaller percentage have a significant fall in insulin dose. Historically, this was attributed to failure of the feto-placental unit. However, there is no association between a fall in insulin requirement and adverse fetal outcome.

– Journal of Obstetric Medicine

Two studies have explored the significance of falling insulin requirements in late gestation. The first, by McManus et al.,50 was a retrospective review of 32 women with T1DM. From 36 weeks until delivery, 62% had a fall in insulin dose.

There were no adverse neonatal outcomes, including in the six women with a more than 15% decrease in insulin dose.

Almost 8% had a fall in insulin requirements of 30% or more within seven days in the third trimester. There was no association with adverse fetal outcome although 61% of these women delivered more than two weeks after the initial decline in insulin. However, the applicability to current practice is debatable as recruitment occurred from 1976 to 1991 and routine induction at 38 weeks was standard practice.

Factors determining insulin requirements in women with type 1 diabetes mellitus during pregnancy: a review. Naomi Achong, corresponding author 1,2 Harold David McIntyre,2, and Leonie Callaway1,2

Despite the evidence of lack of adverse events and a LACK of evidence that falling insulin requirements are an indication for early delivery, the vast majority of doctors will still induce early or do a cesarean, likely just to cover themselves. You may be pressured to induce labor to keep your baby safe, and what mother would argue with that? These mamas will tell the story of their emergency induction or c-section and their failing placenta, when for most of them, the placenta was likely fine.

My take-away here is get checked, monitor the baby, be safe, but don't be bullied into an unnecessary induction or cesarean based only on falling insulin requirements.

Chapter 15: Weeks 37-40

Almost There

Can you believe you are almost there? I'll bet it feels like you have been pregnant forever. You're probably pretty anxious for your baby to get here and excited for the big day. Do you have your birth plan made? Bag packed?

Childcare set up for your other kids if needed? So many things to remember!

What to Pack

You'll want to pack all the regular things for having a baby, as well as all your diabetes supplies. You'll want something comfortable to labor in if you aren't wearing a hospital gown (some mamas buy their own super cute hospital gown to bring with them). You'll want stretchy, comfortable clothes for afterward. An oversized pair of pj's is always a good idea. Bring lots of your preferred pads. The ones the hospital gives you look like they are from 1965 and should require a belt (back before they had pads with adhesive, women had to wear a special "belt" to hold their pad in place). No tampons of course. Some suggest bringing a tennis ball for counter pressure if you experience back labor.

I brought numbing spray in case I tore (boy did I need that!) The hospital gave me some too as well as Preparation H pads which are cooling and decrease swelling. Bring a nursing bra and nursing pads. They'll probably give you Lansinoh to put on your nipples, but I brought my own just in case. I also brought a nursing pillow. This is super helpful if you have a c-section. It will keep the baby's weight off your incision. You might want to bring your own music to listen to during labor. My mom brought me magazines and goodies to distract myself with, but I couldn't focus on any of them because the contractions were so intense.

I wore slippers that looked like flip flops for my second baby because my feet were so swollen. Bring clothes for baby and a coming home outfit. The hospital will provide diapers and wipes. Don't forget socks (for both of you!) I brought hand covers because all my babies scratched themselves. Some people don't like these though. Don't forget some comfortable underwear for afterward. If you had a c-section, you'll definitely want granny panties as low-cut panties will cut into your incision. Ouch! I also brought a back scratcher with #2 because the morphine in the spinal made me itch so badly!

Monitoring after 36 Weeks

Starting at 36 weeks, you'll likely move to twice weekly monitoring and visits (if you aren't already). The doctor might start checking your cervix for dilation around this point also. You can decline these checks if you want as they really don't predict labor, but it is helpful to know how dilated and effaced you are, as well as baby's station (how far down baby is) to know whether an induction is likely to be successful.

Sweeping Membranes

Starting around 37 weeks, your doctor might suggest having your membranes, "swept" or "stripped". This procedure consists of the doctor inserting a gloved finger into your cervix (you need to be at least a fingertip dilated) and sweeping their finger between the membranes of the amniotic sac and your uterus. This releases prostaglandins which could help start labor. Mine also stretched my cervix to dilate me a little more. This process can be uncomfortable but shouldn't be outright painful (though some say it is). It's a very quick procedure.

I had my membranes swept at 37 and 38 weeks (38 and 39 by my dates) and while they started contractions and bloody, "show", they did not start labor.

Supplements

There are various supplements that can be taken to get the body ready for labor. I used Evening Primrose oil orally and vaginally from 35 weeks on, which is supposed to help, "ripen" your cervix and make it more favorable. It does not induce labor. I also drank red raspberry leaf tea, which helps tone your uterus and get it ready for labor. I also used a supplement called 5W which is also supposed to be helpful. Always discuss supplements with your OB/MFM/Midwife. Mine was cool with RRL tea, Evening Primrose Oil and 5W, but warned me not to try castor oil (as I had tried in past pregnancies). Apparently, it can make contractions so intense it can appear on the monitor that the placenta is abrupting.

Natural Induction Methods

If you do a Google search for natural induction methods, you'll find plenty, and I tried most of them! You can try Eggplant Parmigiana, spicy foods, fresh pineapple (be careful with blood sugars), sex (loads of fun when you're as big as a house), walking, nipple stimulation (I used a breast pump), some try castor oil (I don't recommend-gag), and herbal concoctions. They may or may not work. None worked for me unfortunately.

The Big Day

The day you have been waiting for has finally arrived. You are probably excited and terrified. Or maybe you are just ready to be done! You've prepared, you've read all the books, gone to your appointments, packed your bags and you're ready. What should you expect?

We all have a pretty picture of how our birth is going to happen, and most of the time, that picture changes a bit. Not everything in your birth plan happens the way you want it to. Having a healthy baby is the most important thing of course, but this is an important time for you as well. Expect that some things will change but remember to advocate for yourself if things are not going the way they should. You are your biggest advocate.

Author's Story: Aiden's Birth

40 weeks-40 weeks 1 day

My induction was scheduled for Fri, Aug 26, at 5:00. We had decided to induce because of his size (estimated 8lb14oz 2 weeks before). At my Tuesday appointment I was 1-2 cm and 60-70% effaced and was hoping I had made progress.

I went to my Fri appointment at 2:45 and had my final biophysical profile. Everything looked good and I went to do my NST. After a few minutes on the monitor, I got a phone call. It was one of the doctors from L&D and they wanted me to come in early. They said to have the nurse take me off the monitor and to come right to L&D. I was disappointed, as I hadn't eaten and wanted to get dinner before we started. I grabbed an apple and scarfed it down on the way over.

Because of my previous c-sections, we couldn't use Cervidil or Cytotec because of the risk of uterine rupture, so we had decided to try a Foley Bulb induction. Basically, they insert a foley catheter tube into the cervix, and inflate the balloon to manually dilate me to 3 cm or so and then it would fall out. The plan was to leave it overnight and start Pitocin at 8 am. We got there, filled out paperwork and consents, and I got into my gown, started my I.V. and they put me on the monitor.

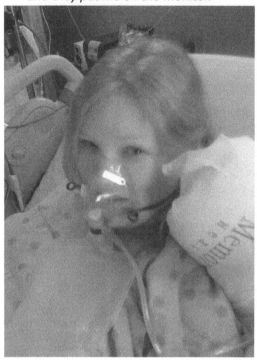

They came in and checked me and I was the same as Tue, 1cm and 60-70% effaced. They inserted the Foley Bulb, and it wasn't too bad, but as soon as the balloon was inflated, I felt intense pressure and had back-to-back strong contractions, almost on top of each other. A little over an hour later, after constant contractions I asked to go to the bathroom. I was told I was not allowed up and could use a bedpan. When I used the bedpan, the Foley Bulb popped out and I couldn't stop going. I also felt this incredible relief from the pressure and contractions. I wondered if my water had broken. The doctor checked me, and my water was indeed broken, and I was dilated to a 4. They immediately started I.V. antibiotics as I was GBS+. I was excited. Things seemed to be progressing quickly.

I continued to contract throughout the night and after my water was broken, they were very intense and painful. The doctors wouldn't check me as my membranes were ruptured and they didn't want to risk infection. By 1 am I was in so much pain I finally caved and asked for an epidural. I had previously said I didn't want one, but I will never again think less of someone for getting one! My spinals with my c-sections were so bad I was terrified, but it was almost painless (probably because I was distracted by the contractions). After getting the epidural, I was able to sleep a little though I didn't get much rest because the baby's heart rate kept dropping and I had to wear an oxygen mask and lie on my left side.

I had this witchy nurse who told me I would have to start an insulin drip and glucose drip once the Pitocin was started. I told her I had already discussed this with my doctor and that he said I could keep my insulin pump and continuous glucose monitor and not have the drips. He had said I could manage my own blood sugars and not be on an ADA diet since I eat lower carb than their recommendations. She said we would see about that.

At 8 am, Dr. Baker came in and checked me. I was 4-5 cm, hardly any progress for all the pain! So glad I got the epi. I asked about keeping my pump and cgm and he said no problem. The nurse didn't say anything. They started the Pitocin and within an hour or so I was at 7 cm, and 100% effaced. After another hour I was at 9 and at -1. By this point my epidural had stopped working on my left side, but nobody acted like they believed me. I felt every contraction but only on the left.

Around 1 they checked me, and I was complete and +1. Plus one refers to the baby's station. "An imaginary line is drawn between the two bones in the pelvis (known as ischial spines). This is the "zero" line, and when the baby reaches this line it is considered to be in "zero station." When the baby is above this imaginary line it is in a minus station. When the baby is below, it is in a "plus" station. Stations are measured from -5 at the pelvic inlet to +4 at the pelvic outlet." I was told I could start pushing soon. I was really excited and ready to go.

A few minutes later the doctor comes in and says he wants to wait until I am at +2. I was so disappointed. It wasn't long though that I was checked again and told I was at +2. One of the residents came in and said we would start pushing. I was freaking out at this point because Matt had gone outside thinking we had plenty of time. I called him and he was just down the hall

thank goodness. The doctors told me to go ahead and push. I gave a good push and she's like "stop"! She gets on the phone and tells Dr Baker if he wants to deliver me, he better get in there.

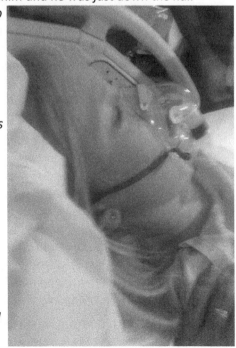

Dr. Baker comes in with a bunch of other doctors (later I found out various years of residents and med students). I guess vba2c is pretty rare and they wanted to watch. They had me wait until the very peak of a contraction and then push. This was crazy hard as I had this incredible urge to push and pushing made the pain better. After a couple rounds of pushing someone told me to reach down and touch my baby's head. It was the most surreal experience. A couple more pushes and he was out!

They let me lift him up on my chest and I immediately started bawling. I couldn't believe I was holding my baby and I had actually done it! I got my VBAC. I really didn't think it was going to happen until he was actually out. The doctor had gone on about how big the baby was and how he might get stuck. I prayed over and over for God to please not let me rupture and to protect my baby. They let Matt cut the cord and I got to snuggle with Adrian for an hour before they took him. I was so thrilled.

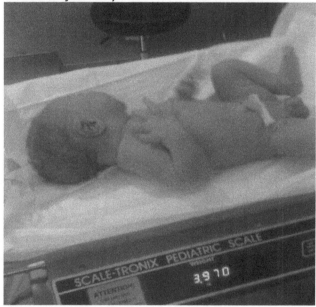

The doctors and nurses were taking bets on how big he was. Everyone said over 9lb. He was 8lb12oz (2 oz less than the estimate 2 weeks before!) and 21.5 inches long. I did tear pretty badly. It was only 2nd degree, but I tore every which way. It took over an hour to stitch me up and the doctor told me he had never used that many sutures on a repair. I didn't care though. I was on a high. It was the most amazing experience of my life.

I am so grateful that I got this experience. I really feel like I got the healing birth that I longed for. Just about every nurse commented on my "extensive repair" and asked if I wish I had just gotten the c-section. I say most definitely not! The difference in recovery is like night and day. I was feeling great and up and around in a couple hours. I was eating and wearing my own pajamas. We are now 3 days postpartum, and things are going great! He nurses like a pro and I am recovering well. We did have to stay 48 hours because my water had been broken for so long and I was GBS+ but everything was fine. Adrian and Daddy are already good buddies. Matt can get him to stop crying every time.

* Edited to add: my blood sugars stayed between 70-125 the entire time and Adrian did not have any low blood sugars as I was told he would (ha-ha).

Induction

Bishop's Score

Is your body ready for an induction? Is your cervix favorable? Is an induction likely to be successful? A Bishop's Score can help predict this. It is based on the position of your cervix. Is your cervix anterior (nearer the opening of the vagina) or posterior (farther away)? Is your cervix firm or soft? A firm cervix will feel kind of like the tip of your nose. A firm cervix is more resistant to stretching. How effaced is your cervix? Effacement is the measurement of how thick or thin your cervix is. A normal cervix is usually about 3cm long, whereas a fully effaced cervix will be paper thin. How dilated are you? Dilation is the measurement of how open your cervix is. Your cervix needs to dilate to 10cm to deliver a baby and if you have already started to dilate and efface, induction will likely be more successful. When I was induced, I was at 1-2 cm with 60-70% effacement. My cervix was soft and anterior. This gave me a score of 7.

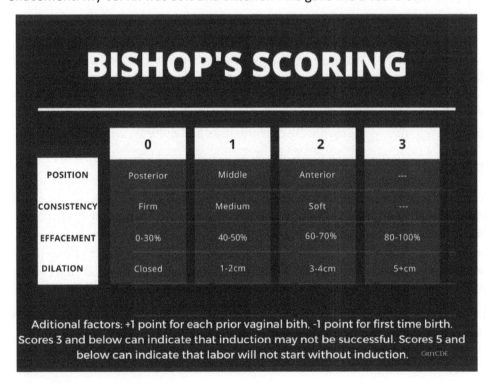

BISHOP'S SCORING

	0	1	2	3
POSITION	Posterior	Middle	Anterior	---
CONSISTENCY	Firm	Medium	Soft	---
EFFACEMENT	0-30%	40-50%	60-70%	80-100%
DILATION	Closed	1-2cm	3-4cm	5+cm

Aditional factors: +1 point for each prior vaginal bith, -1 point for first time birth. Scores 3 and below can indicate that induction may not be successful. Scores 5 and below can indicate that labor will not start without induction. GRITCDE

Prostaglandin Gel

If your cervix isn't favorable, your doctor might have you come in the night before and use prostaglandin gel or a vaginal insert called Cervidil, which helps to 'ripen' your cervix by making it softer.

Foley Bulb

The doctor will insert a Foley Catheter into your cervix, and then inflate the balloon with saline to mechanically dilate your cervix. For me, as soon as the balloon was inflated, I felt immense pressure and back-to-back contractions.

When the balloon falls out, you'll likely be around 3-4cm and your water can be broken. Mine broke on its own when the balloon came out.

Amniotomy

Your doctor will use a special tool that looks kind of like a crochet hook, called an amnihook to artificially rupture your membranes, thereby breaking your water and starting labor. Contractions are much more intense once the membranes are ruptured.

Cytotec

The medication Misoprostol or Cytotec is a prostaglandin medication that may be used to induce labor. Misoprostol can be given orally, sublingually, or vaginally. In studies, it showed to be more effective at producing delivery within 24 hours, but with the risk of uterine hyperstimulation and the risk of uterine rupture. Though it is not FDA approved for the induction of labor, many doctors are comfortable using it. If you have had a previous cesarean section, it's not a good idea to use Misoprostol. Discuss the risks and benefits with your doctor.

Pitocin

The synthetic form of the hormone oxytocin, which is the hormone that causes labor to start naturally, is the most commonly used medication for induction of labor. It can cause intense contractions, and if the dose is too high, can cause uterine hyperstimulation or put the baby in distress, so it should be given in small doses with close monitoring. The use of Pitocin often necessitates the need for an epidural, which in some women, can slow down labor.

I was given Pitocin after I stalled at 5 cm after 15 hours of labor. It worked pretty well, though at some points we had to slow down the rate, and I had to turn on my left side and wear an oxygen mask, because Adrian's heart rate was decelerating.

Unmedicated Birth/Going into Labor Naturally

This can be difficult to accomplish as a t1, but it can be done! My hat's off to the mamas who pull this off. Make your intentions clear beforehand, and don't let yourself be pressured into something you aren't comfortable with.

There are alternatives to traditional medicated labors, such as having a saline lock in place in case of emergency and using alternative pain relief measures such as Hypnobabies or a TENS unit.

Home Birth

A rare few type 1 mamas have had home births. This is definitely not something that is without risk and most midwives won't take on type 1's, especially for a home birth due to the risks of things like macrosomia causing shoulder dystocia or baby getting 'stuck'. This is a decision that should not be made lightly. Take all factors into consideration, keeping in mind that if blood sugars are not absolutely normal, this is a pretty big risk. How fast can the midwife get there? How close are you to the hospital? Will there be monitoring in case the baby goes into distress?

With my third baby, I had fallen off the wagon pretty hard regarding carbohydrate intake. MyA1C's were between 5.9 and 6.5. However, I had decided to try for a home birth this time. (Disclaimer: I am not advocating for attempting a home birth with anything higher than non-diabetic-range blood sugars but am just telling my story.) I figured that I had one vaginal birth already and got an epidural but never needed Pitocin. It was not hard to find three midwives who would have taken me, here in Florida, as long as they were not responsible for the diabetes part, which I assured them they would not be. The midwife I chose consulted with an OB who approved that I was not too high of a risk. She said she had never had an "emergency transfer" during labor- she always saw early warning signs and transferred her clients to OB's before labor began. There was also a maternity hospital 7 minutes from my house, so I felt confident that if an emergency arose, help was close by. Labor started on its own early in the morning 1 day past my due date. As before I did not have a CGM or pump but took half my normal long-acting insulin and checked my blood sugar a handful of times throughout. My midwife encouraged me to eat but I did not feel like eating. Labor started on its own, but as slowly as before. After 39 hours of labor, I was at about 5 cm and I was feeling so discouraged and exhausted and in pain that I told them I might want to go to the hospital for an epidural. My midwife encouraged me to take a magnesium drink and wait an hour, so I agreed. Shortly after that I felt my body pushing uncontrollably. My midwife came into the room and felt the baby's head! It took 39 hours to get from 1cm to 5cm but less than an hour to go from 5cm to 10 and crowning!

His head was out with one push but then his shoulders seemed to be stuck. My midwife had me change positions (I had been sitting on the toilet, so she had me sit on the bed with my legs pulled back) and the rest of him came out. He was blue and making squeaky noises but not yet breathing. The cord had not been cut, so he was still getting oxygen that way, but it had been temporarily cut off when the cord was pinched as he came out. The midwife gave him a couple puffs of air and he soon let out a big scream.

She did not test his blood sugar, but she stayed for 4 hours after the birth and he had no low blood sugar symptoms. He weighed 10 lbs. even, I believe due to my much higher carb intake, but I only had a tiny tear this time and did not require stitches. My natural birth was by far the most painful during labor but also the easiest, quickest recovery. My son had a lip and tongue tie that hampered breastfeeding at first and we supplemented but after it was revised, we were able to get to solely breastfeeding for over a year.

- Katherine Witherell

Pain Relief

I.V. Pain Relief

There are a few options for pain relief during labor. I.V. (intravenous) medication such as Nubain or Stadol is one option. I tried this first, but it made me feel 'loopy' and I really didn't like it. It didn't do much for pain. Some women find it helpful to "take the edge off" though. I.V. medication does have the potential to cross the placenta and make your baby sleepy, which some moms want to avoid.

Transcutaneous Electrical Nerve Stimulation (TENS)

Some women find a TENS very effective during labor. It's not very popular in the U.S. and is used more often in Canada and the U.K. but it is a low-risk option that some mamas swear by. A TENS unit is a small device that has electrodes connected to it that stick to your skin (kind of like an EKG) which deliver a mild electrical current which can interrupt the pain signal or possibly cause your body to release endorphins (natural pain killers). It feels kind of like a buzzing or like 'crawling' on your skin. It's a very safe option and is available fairly inexpensively on Amazon.

Hypnosis

Another method of pain relief that isn't used too often is self-hypnosis, such as, "Hypnobabies". This option is more popular with the natural birth crowd who prefer to avoid medications during labor.

Nitrous Oxide

This is yet another option that is not very popular in the United States. In the U.K. it's commonly known as 'gas and air (50% nitrous oxide and 50% oxygen)'. Nitrous oxide is a gas that is delivered through a mask. You may have had experience with it during dental procedures.

It can be an effective form of pain relief and can be used as needed. You place the mask over your face as you are having a contraction and take it off once it has ended. The effects are fast and wear off rather quickly once it is removed. It has few side effects and if you do have any (dizziness or nausea for instance) they wear off quickly).

Epidural

This is by far the most popular form of pain relief during labor in the United States. A thin plastic catheter is inserted into the epidural space in your lower spine through which medication is delivered which will numb you from your abdomen down. In many hospitals, you'll be given a button to push to control the amount of medication given.

I personally was terrified of having an epidural, as I had negative experience with spinal anesthesia during my C-sections. I was determined to have all-natural labor and was very annoyed at the nurses and doctors who I felt were pressuring me into getting one. However, after 10 grueling hours of intense contractions, I was exhausted and gave in.

All my fears were for naught. I was so distracted by the contractions that I didn't feel a thing. The hardest part was having to curl up and arch my back. The area will be cleaned and numbed with a local anesthetic, then a needle will be inserted to introduce the catheter. The needle will then be removed and the catheter left in place and taped down, like an I.V..

After the epidural is started, you'll likely have a Foley catheter inserted into your bladder. It won't hurt as you'll be numb. An 'in and out' catheter may be used as an alternative. My Foley Catheter was removed when it was time to start pushing.

There are downsides to an epidural. Obviously, your mobility will be limited and you won't be able to change positions easily. You'll also be out on a continuous fetal monitor if you weren't already on one. It is possible that an epidural will slow your labor, which could make a cesarean more likely.

During Labor

Insulin needs tend to decrease during labor as your body is working hard and those who do MDI may need to reduce their long-acting insulin if you aren't on an insulin drip.

Those pumping can switch to a temp basal as needed. Your blood sugar will typically be checked every 4 hours, but I was checking much more frequently on my Dexcom. The nurses just let me tell them my Dexcom reading instead of poking my finger, so that was nice. Do make sure your Dexcom is reading accurately beforehand. When I got to the point of pushing, the doctor would ask for a bg reading every few minutes and the nurse would yell it out to him. It may be helpful to have liquid glucose on hand to treat lows as it works very rapidly, and sometimes nurses can respond slowly.

Cesarean Section

There are many reasons you might end up with a c-section. Don't ignore this portion of the book just because you think you won't have one. I made that mistake and regretted it immensely. You may end up with a c-section if your labor fails to progress, if you have placenta previa, if you have preeclampsia, if you have proliferative retinopathy, if your baby is in distress, if your baby is breech, transverse, if you have a multiple gestation and many other reasons.

A cesarean isn't the end of the world, and it is much more common to have a family centered, 'gentle' cesarean nowadays, which can make the process much better. A 'gentle' cesarean involves being able to witness the delivery of the baby, either by lowering the drape or by having a clear drape. Baby is placed on mom's chest and breastfeeding right away is encouraged. Mom and baby are kept together as much as possible. This method would have made things so much better for me.

For a c-section, you'll generally be given spinal anesthesia. In some cases, usually if you were previously in labor, an epidural will be used. A spinal, also known as a subarachnoid block, is an injection into the subarachnoid space in your spine which will make you numb from the abdomen down. While you're having your spinal, your partner will likely have to leave the room, but will be brought back in after the spinal.

After this, you'll be laid on the operating table and a Foley Catheter will be inserted into your bladder. Make sure to ask them to insert it *after* your spinal so you don't feel it. It's much nicer that way. After this your abdomen will be cleaned with a special solution. You won't feel anything when the doctor makes the incision into your abdomen and your uterus. You'll feel a lot of pressure, as well as pulling and tugging. With my daughter (my breech baby) it felt like someone was sitting on my abdomen. There was so much pressure getting her out. If you can, keep your pump on for the c-section if you use one. I was able to keep mine with my first baby, and everything went very smoothly. I wasn't allowed to wear it with my second and it was awful. Be sure to wear it somewhere that won't get in the way of your incision. You can wear it on your arm but be sure they don't put your blood pressure cuff on that arm. You can also use your hip (that's what I did) or upper thigh.

After the baby is out, they'll deliver your placenta and close you back up. In many cases, your baby will be placed on your chest (note in your birth plan if you want this done). Baby will be checked out and given an APGAR score based on color, breathing, crying, and tone. Baby will be weighed and cleaned up and blood sugar will be measured to make sure your baby isn't hypoglycemic.

After you are closed up, you'll go to the recovery room to be monitored. Find out if you will be allowed to have your baby with you in recovery. With my second c-section, I wasn't allowed to keep my baby in the room because none of the recovery nurses were certified in infant CPR. This was very upsetting.

After your c-section, your doctor won't want you lying in bed all the time. Once you are able to get up, you'll be encouraged to walk around to prevent blood clots and pneumonia. This can be a very unpleasant experience. It can be hard to stand up because you feel like your incision will rip open. Bracing a pillow against your incision can be helpful, as well as walking with the baby cart to use like a 'walker'. Getting up and walking as quickly as possible can help immensely with recovery.

Be sure to ask for pain medications if you need them and ask before the pain is too intense. Some women have a lot of pain, and others have very little.

Everything was great. I wouldn't change one thing. They asked what music I liked and played Maroon 5 in the OR. They delayed cord clamping and after being checked out was on my chest the whole time. We tried breast feeding. Despite some low BGs the first day or two, he was with me the whole time. I had zero pain from the c-section - the whole thing was great. As soon as I had feeling back, I was walking, showering, using the bathroom, getting in and out of bed, getting the baby in and out of his bassinet, walking the halls with him. The nurses were great. No issues at all.

-Kerri Martin

My diabetes journey started shortly before my first pregnancy. I was diagnosed with Type 2 diabetes at 22 years of age (but my diagnosis was later changed to Type 1). My husband and I had been trying to conceive for about 7 months without success. As soon as my blood sugars were closer to normal range (diagnosed with an a1c of 12.6 and blood sugar of 1000mg/dL) I got pregnant (with an A1c of 7.6).

My first pregnancy was reasonably well-controlled on a mostly standard American diet, but I still did count and limit carbs to some extent. My A1c's stayed between 5.9 and 6.2. My OB only wanted me to check my blood sugar 4 times a day and take insulin at dinner without testing. He also wanted me to call in every evening and leave a message with my blood sugars that day. However, his nurse called back one time and wanted me to change my insulin-take more without testing first, after just one high reading, without looking at the trend! He and my endo got into an argument over the phone and my endo almost fired himself from my case, but I was able to convince my OB to just worry about standard pregnancy stuff and to let my endo handle my diabetes. I typically tested my blood sugar about 6-8 times a day.

My OB was very nervous letting a diabetic go to term and convinced me to induce, but I pushed him to just 2 days before my due date. I really wanted a home birth all along, but I figured it was too risky for a diabetic. I still wanted as natural a birth as possible, so I breast pump my way into labor and took a small amount of castor oil, and labor really took off, even though I was walking and moving the whole time. I did not test my blood sugar consistently during labor and I did not have a pump or CGM. I did take half my normal long-acting insulin, but I didn't eat or take other insulin while in the hospital. My OB's midwife was attending, and she broke my water and there was meconium (baby's first poop) in the water-not good. The midwife knew I did not want Pitocin so she never pushed it, but looking back, since labor never took off on its own, (I stayed 3 cm all day, about 15 hours), I should have consented to it. In the end, they said my baby was in distress and did a c-section (which they later wrote down as, "failure to progress"). My baby girl did have a fever at birth, and they kept her in the hospital 7 days on antibiotics, but it was not related to my diabetes. They had estimated her weight to be about 8lb. before birth, but she was born at 7lb. even. She was breast feeding great until they gave her bottles in the NICU, but after we got back home again, she did great breast feeding for over a year.

-Katherine Witherell

Insulin needs can drop pretty quickly after delivery, though for me, it was not right away. It was more like the next morning. I was instructed to cut my basals in half the next morning, which worked pretty well. If you wear a cgm, this will be very helpful in determining when you need to decrease your insulin. If you are on MDI, splitting basal can help a lot, not just because of gaps in coverage, but because you can make changes more quickly.

After Delivery

Once the baby is delivered, he or she will be assessed and assigned an APGAR score which is based on baby's appearance, pulse, grimace, activity, and respiration. This can all be done while your baby is lying on your chest in most cases. This assessment is done at one minute and five minutes after birth. Your doctor will likely also inject some Pitocin into your I.V. bag or give you an intramuscular shot of Pitocin to get your uterus to continue contracting to get back to its normal size. If you delivered vaginally, you'll likely feel the urge to push again when your placenta is being delivered. This is not painful. You might also decide whether you want your placenta to be delivered naturally. Many doctors will apply traction to remove the placenta more quickly.

APGAR SCORING

	INDICATOR	0 POINTS	1 POINT	2 POINTS
A	Appearance	Blue; Pale	Pink body; Blue extremities	Pink
P	Pulse	Absent	<100 bom	>100 bpm
G	Grimace	Floppy	Minimal response to stimulation	Prompt response to stimulation
A	Activity	Absent	Flexed Arms & Legs	Active
R	Respiration	Absent	Slow and Irregular	Vigorous Cry

GRITCDE

After this, your baby will be given an antibiotic eye antibiotic ointment and a shot of Vitamin K (to help blood clotting) in its thigh. This process is sometimes referred to as, 'eyes and thighs'. The ointment is to prevent blindness caused by bacteria in the birth canal. These can also be done while baby is on your chest if everything checks out health wise. You can put your preferences on this in your birth plan in addition to whether you want the umbilical cord clamped (this is typically done one minute after birth, but some wish to let baby get all its blood back, so they wait until the cord has stopped pulsating). Do your research on the risks and benefits of this. Some t1 mamas may decide to bank their child's cord blood for the future so this is also something to take into consideration.

Baby will be weighed and measured at some point during all this. I requested to wait an hour with my baby on my chest before doing these. You, your partner, and your baby will all receive matching bracelets, soon after birth as well for security. Baby's blood sugar will be tested as type 1 moms often have babies with hypoglycemia. This practice is happening more and more even with non-diabetic moms. This heel-stick blood sugar can be done with your baby in the room with you. Find out hospital protocols in regard to all these before your birth so you can make your birth plan the way you want it and there are no surprises.

If you've had a vaginal delivery, you will be assessed for tears and will be stitched up if needed. I barely remember this as I was busy snuggling my baby. You can go ahead and try to nurse your baby, but don't worry if your baby doesn't latch right away. Babies aren't hungry right away. During this time and over the next few hours, (whether you've had a vaginal delivery or a c-section) a nurse will apply pressure to your abdomen, known as 'fundal massage'. This is done to get your uterus back down to its normal size and is a bit uncomfortable, but necessary.

Neonatal Hypoglycemia

What if your baby's blood sugar is low? In a neonate (newborn) hypoglycemia is defined as a blood glucose less than 45mg/dL (2.5mmol/L). I know that sounds ridiculously low, but babies run a good bit lower (a good thing to remember if you worried about lows hurting the baby). Neonatal hypoglycemia can happen if mom's blood sugar has been on the higher side (some studies show above 110mg/dL (6.1 mmol/L) at birth leads to a higher risk of baby being hypo).

Prematurity is a higher risk for hypoglycemia, and sometimes it just happens regardless of blood sugar control. Maternal blood sugars can be beautiful, and baby still ends up low.

Some moms want to avoid formula and bottles. What is the solution? Many mamas collect their colostrum (pre-milk) in syringes and freeze it to bring to the hospital in case baby has low blood sugar.

Baby can be given dextrose (sugar water) if necessary and can be fed through a syringe rather than a bottle. Formula is NOT necessary!

Jaundice

Sometimes babies of diabetic moms are jaundiced. This means that your baby's bilirubin levels are elevated, which causes the skin, and the whites of the eyes to be yellow. As discussed earlier, this is caused by extra red blood cells being present, which elevate bilirubin levels when broken down. Why is this an issue? Because very high levels of bilirubin can affect your baby's nervous system or brain.

Jaundice is corrected with a special blanket or light that your baby is put under to lower the bilirubin levels. Feeding will also speed up the elimination of bilirubin, so mamas are often pressured into using formula. Many times, phototherapy is enough, and formula is not needed. Breastfeeding needs to be frequent and effective to eliminate jaundice. If formula is needed, you can ask for your baby to be fed using a spoon, cup, or eyedropper if you don't wish a bottle to be used.

Chapter 16: Grit Pregnancy Testimonials

I manage two pregnancy groups on Facebook for pregnant diabetics. Grit Pregnancies is a group for pregnant diabetic women (any kind) who eat low carb and follow Dr. Bernstein's guidelines. This group has had such amazing results. Babies are healthy, normal sized and full-term, without all the complications we see in typical diabetic pregnancies. Positive Type One Diabetic Pregnancies is a mainstream group for type 1 diabetic pregnant mommies. I was a member of this group before I was an admin and these ladies helped me through 2 pregnancies. It's a great resource. I'd like to share some of their stories.

Success Stories

On Audrey

I became pregnant with my daughter at age 27, in 2016, as a graduate student. At the time, I had already been eating a low-carbohydrate diet for about a year. My first A1c during the pregnancy was 5.7%, and later on, lingered between 5.1-5.2% for the duration of the pregnancy.

I focused on getting ample protein, like eggs, chicken, beef, and fish, as well as a large amount of nutrient-dense, non-starchy vegetables. For snacks, I focused on high-calorie, low-carb options, like nuts and cheese, veggies dipped in peanut butter or dip, as well as more fancy items like seaweed and cream cheese roll-ups with smoked salmon. I often prepared low-carb cloud bread and Swedish buns in lieu of grain alternatives.

Throughout, I carefully monitored my blood glucose levels with the help of a continuous glucose monitor and made frequent adjustments to my basal and bolus insulin doses (I used Levemir, split twice per day, and Humalog for meals and corrections).

At 20 weeks pregnant, I moved cross-country and had to switch providers. I got some push-back from the new maternal-fetal-medicine (MFM) team because I refused to go to their pregnancy clinic and be followed by an endocrinologist. I chose to manage all my own insulin adjustments and only saw them for ultrasounds and the delivery.

Over time, and with additional reassurance of scan after scan indicating a very healthy pregnancy, the relationship with the new healthcare team became less strained. They began to be more open to treating me as an individual.

When we learned that my daughter was stubbornly breech, and I opted against having her turned, they even agreed to schedule my c-section for 40 weeks and 2 ways, which is exceedingly rare for someone with type 1 diabetes.

I went into spontaneous labor at 39 weeks and 4 days, and my daughter was born via c-section the next morning. Everything went smoothly. She weighed 6 lb. 11 oz. and scored perfectly on both of her APGAR tests. She never left my side, did not have low blood sugar levels or jaundice, and was exclusively breastfed for almost one year.

One issue I had was with the hospital protocol of having an insulin/glucose drip. As I feared, the team was following an algorithm for dosing that likely would have killed me had they not broken the rules (upon my advice) of disconnecting me shortly after delivery. The algorithm was reactive (based on fingerstick blood glucose levels), but I knew that after delivery, insulin needs drop very dramatically. When I saw that I was 70 mg/dL and trending downward several hours after delivery, I insisted that they disconnect the drip (I still had Levemir working in my system, too).

I had an uncomplicated C-section recovery, and vowed that for my next baby, I would demand to be in control of my diabetes management throughout my delivery and hospital stay."

-Maria Muccioli, PhD, Diabetes Daily

During my first pregnancy I was diagnosed with gestational diabetes. I immediately switched to a low carb diet in an effort to control my blood glucose. Low-carb just intuitively made sense to me. If I had a disease that made processing sugar problematic, I should limit all sources of it.

Being new to diabetes management, I was not well versed in using insulin, which I quickly needed, or aware of the implications of even slightly elevated numbers during pregnancy. While my control at the time was not as tight as it was with my second pregnancy, the low carb diet surely kept my numbers from spiraling radically out of control. My son was born premature, but did not suffer from blood sugar problems, and was completely healthy. What a blessing!

Fast forward to three months after his birth, I was in the hospital in diabetic ketoacidosis, and formally diagnosed with type 1 diabetes the following week. For the next few months, I tried to manage on a typical diet, closer to a paleo approach, with limited sweets and slower acting carbs. Things weren't working. The low blood sugars which I experienced following high carb meals (even "healthy carbs" like beans, lentils, or fruit) with rapid acting insulin were terrifying. I finally decided to buckle down and commit to a diet of 20 carbs or less per day and avoided any foods that caused me problems. I learned to replicate all my favorites with low carb options. Who knew turnips were so great at replacing classics like scalloped potatoes on Easter?

By the time I became pregnant with my second child, about two years later, my A1C was down to 5.4%. I was down to my lowest weight in about five years and felt wonderful. My pregnancy proceeded beautifully, weight gain was minimal, and I had a perfectly healthy full-term baby girl with no unnecessary interventions. The labor went smoothly, even with eating meals, and plenty of insulin on-board throughout.

I was able to consistently keep my A1C below 5% without suffering from debilitating low blood sugars or rapid blood sugar spikes. Sure, management changed from day to day, and I had to make plenty of adjustments frequently, that's just the nature of being diabetic during pregnancy.

What made it doable was my consistent low carb meals. Even if I had a "bad day," with numbers rising unexpectedly, I could manage. I never felt deprived either. During the dreaded weeks of nausea from morning sickness, I got by with plenty of almond flour scones to fill up my stomach and bone broth to keep me hydrated.

Today I feel completely empowered by going through pregnancy, delivery, and postpartum with my diabetes. I wish all diabetics could experience the peace of knowing food is not the enemy. If you take out the biggest factor, the foods that are difficult for us to process (those that are high in carbohydrate), insulin management is so much easier. The high blood sugar numbers aren't really too high, not usually above 140 at most. If a low blood sugar happens, it is slower in its fall rate, and not as severe. An added benefit of the low carb lifestyle is that you feel and look great!

Pregnancy is scary enough, managing with a low carb diet made the experience a joyful one. I wasn't sure if I would ever want another pregnancy when I first found out I was pregnant with my daughter. I had serious and well-founded fears about my diabetes and its implications on the baby. I can honestly say, I wouldn't hesitate to do it again. I know I can have what any other non-diabetic woman can, a smooth pregnancy and healthy baby. All diabetics deserve to have healthy blood sugars and low carb can make that a reality."

-Megan Kelly

I was diagnosed at age 30 and had my first child at 36. My intention was to have a natural, vaginal birth with minimal interventions. I wanted to work with midwives and the hospital/midwife practice with the best rates and most vaginal delivery/breastfeeding friendly reputation, is a teaching hospital near me. It took a lot of negotiation, educating and advocating for myself, but I convinced the midwives to help birth my baby. My philosophy was that given my level of health, excellent a1c, that I would take the normal tests of any mom and if the tests showed anything to be concerned about, we'd follow up with additional tests. I turned down many of the standard additional tests that they usually give diabetics just for being diabetic.

I knew that I wanted to have a minimum-intervention birth and I was really hoping that it would be a natural, vaginal birth. I had attended ICAN meetings (International Cesarean Awareness Network) meetings in my area when I was planning to conceive, and it was heartbreaking to hear about the experiences these women had with their babies' births. So many people are pressured or scared into having cesarean births and have negative feelings or trauma associated with their labor and delivery. I knew, as a type 1 diabetic, there was a possibility that I could fall prey to the same fate. When I searched the web and read books about pregnancy and type 1 diabetes, it seemed like the majority of these women had cesarean births and/or were pressured into doing inductions, which often cascaded into a cesarean birth. I decided that I really wanted to give birth with midwives, but I couldn't find any midwives in my area that were willing to work with a type 1 diabetic. I did find a doula who had a lot of experience, including with women with type 1 diabetes and she thought my best bet would be at a local teaching hospital that had a good midwifery program.

Due to a low carbohydrate and healthy diet and very close attention to my blood sugars, including with a Dexcom continuous glucose monitor, I was able to maintain A1Cs from 4.8 to 5.2 throughout my pregnancy. I was also very healthy, even for a 35-year-old "geriatric" mother. The OBs I met with all felt that even though my blood sugar was similar to a normal, healthy person, and the fact that I was able to control my autoimmune antibodies with certain protocols, the OBs felt that there was something inherent about the diabetes that put me at high risk and therefore, the OBs insisted they would be in charge of my care. I pushed and pushed on this. I mentioned research, I suggested the OBs look into Dr. Lois Jovanovich and the success she had with Type 1 diabetic mothers.

Finally, we negotiated that if I went into labor naturally (not having to be induced) and there were no medical emergencies, I would be able to give birth with the midwives. The midwives were themselves, a bit nervous about this as they had never made an exception to their rule to NOT work with insulin-dependent diabetics. I assured them that I would manage my own blood sugar, I wanted the same type of birth that they promoted, and it would all be fine! It was a huge accomplishment to come to this agreement and it did not happen without a LOT of stressful meetings with certain OBs who were very nasty and fear mongering. I walked away from at least two appointments completely in tears. But in the end, it was all worth it.

I went into labor two days prior to my due date. I was walking a lot, having sex, and doing acupuncture to avoid the need for an induction, which I had agreed to consider in week 41. When I went into labor, my doula had assured me that the baby was going to come right away --perhaps even in the car, so imagine my surprise when we arrived at the hospital and they felt that I was still in early labor! I hadn't had any sleep the prior night due to my contractions and that second night in the hospital, I didn't sleep either. The timing of my contractions was all over the place. It turns out that the baby was asynclitic and there was a nuchal arm. My baby's hand was on her face, causing her elbow to obstruct the passage, plus the long side of her head was trying to pass through the more narrow part of the birth canal.

Thankfully, because the midwives are very patient and do not have timelines. 36 hours after my contractions started, my water broke, and I began pushing. I also pushed for 4 hours. It was towards the end of that time that they discovered the nuchal arm/elbow issue, and the skilled midwife was able to slip my baby's hand to the other side of her head, tucking in her elbow, and the baby flew out! Yes, it required some patience, but it was a painless experience, I managed to have a non-medicated vaginal birth and left feeling supported by the hospital staff and very empowered.

-Amelia Kissick

I felt in control and felt informed of all the options presented. I feel lucky that my induction went so quickly for a first-time mother. I started Cytotec at 9pm and was able to stop taking it by 5am the next day as I was contracting regularly on my own. At 9am the foley bulb was taken out and I progressed enough to start Pitocin. Pitocin was titrated up until around 1:30pm when I was fully dilated and ready to push. Dilation happened very quickly once Pitocin started. I pushed for just under two hours, had minimal tearing, and managed labor without any pain medication.

I self-managed my diabetes and never rose above 110. I wore a Dexcom and insulin pump, and the hospital also tested my blood sugar frequently *during the pushing stage (although I have no recollection of this). When I began contracting more regularly overnight, I reduced my basal by 25% on my insulin pump. By morning I reduced to 50%, and when Pitocin started kicking in, I suspended my pump. I kept my pump suspended until 2 hours after delivery, at the direction of the hospital endocrine team. There's only one thing I regret during my birth experience, and that is listening to the endocrine team. I was advised to let my blood sugar rise to at least 200mg/dL before turning my pump off (a number I hadn't reached in over a year!). I trusted them as I didn't know how my body would react post-baby. It took my 20+ hours to get my blood sugar back down and in normal range.*

My birth GOALS were to go pain med free (no epidural), and to have the least amount of interventions as possible (beyond Pitocin). I am very happy with my birth and the ability to follow my goals"

-Leah Wornath

This is the story of how Scarlett Alexandra Youngblood was born! I'm actually going to start with some things that I did during pregnancy which I believe made my pregnancy, labor, and delivery so healthy and successful.

I have had type 1 diabetes for almost 28 years. In the years leading up to trying to conceive, I switched OB/GYN practices. I was frustrated that my HbA1Cs were not in the ideal pregnancy range (less than 6.5%), and I wasn't being given adequate guidance by my endocrinologist.

I took the nutrition classes in the spring of 2016 targeting insulin resistance, which reinforced what I already knew about achieving nondiabetic blood sugar control from the book "Dr. Bernstein's Diabetes Solution" - carbohydrates needed to go. I quickly adopted a low carb diet, avoiding all grains, legumes, starchy vegetables, and fruits 90% of the time I ate, and within 3 months, my HbA1C was 6.3%. It remained in the low 6s, and even dipped into the high 5% range, for the next three years.

We did pretty extensive testing after my two miscarriages in late 2018 to see if there was a culprit that we were unaware of. I had been taking thyroid medication for hypothyroidism since 2010, but that disorder had developed one step further into Hashimoto's Thyroiditis, the autoimmune version of hypothyroidism. With many tweaks to medications and consults with my endocrinologist and OB/GYN, we were given the green light to try to get pregnant again in late spring 2019. By mid-summer, this little lady was on her way!

Besides the fact that my main food groups during pregnancy were protein, fat, and non-starchy vegetables, as well as some store-bought "keto" and "paleo" products, the other thing that I was incredibly consistent with was exercise. I took my first trimester pretty easy, going for short walks, bike rides, and doing yoga on YouTube when I had the energy. Once I hit 14 weeks, I began attending classes again. Barre is such a safe and healthy workout for pregnancy! It has been my go-to form of exercise when I need something that is time efficient and effective, and I knew it would be the perfect thing for me during pregnancy. I attended 4-5 classes in the studio per week from 14 weeks through 38 weeks and added other prenatal workout videos or walks on other days. I would have gone to class during the week of my induction if it hadn't been for the Coronavirus!

Because I really focused on eating high quality, nutritious food, eating to hunger and not counting calories or eating in excess, minimizing my insulin use as much as possible, and working out 5-6 days a week, I only gained 15 pounds. I never felt uncomfortable or taxed, and I loved every minute of being pregnant.

It was predicted that my total daily insulin use through my pump would double by the end of my pregnancy. At its peak, I was taking about 1.5 times my pre-pregnancy dose, and that even tapered off over the last 4 weeks of the pregnancy to about 1.25 times.

I received extra monitoring in my 3rd trimester since my pregnancy was considered high risk. I had consistent biophysical profiles, as well as non-stress tests. It is common and possible for babies born to moms with type 1 to be big babies. This is called macrosomia. Sometimes this means preterm labor, and baby's lungs aren't developed yet. But we were never concerned with that for me and the peanut, based on my growth ultrasounds.

Even though I kept incredible tight control, I couldn't limit all out-of-range blood sugars. My average HbA1C throughout my pregnancy was 5.5% - for reference, someone is considered "prediabetic" with an HbA1C of 5.7%.

Even though I was living with non-diabetic blood sugar levels, we still wanted to make sure baby girl was thriving, and my placenta was doing its job. Because of this risk, my doctors had always told me that we would schedule an induction at 39 weeks instead of waiting for spontaneous labor to start.

Some of you may be wondering why I wasn't just scheduled for a C-section. First of all, healing from major surgery would be much more taxing for someone with diabetes. Second of all, on my first meeting with Dr. Cavallo, the main provider at the practice, he told me that it was his goal for me to have a vaginal delivery. Any way in which we could help my daughter's immune system was a goal we both had, and delivery is one way to do that.

Around 36.5 weeks, I started having noticeable contractions that registered on the non-stress test monitor. That was exciting for me! I was terrified that I would get to my induction date and my body just wouldn't be ready to give birth. Thankfully, that wasn't the case. I continued to have contractions, though nothing consistent, and when we walked into the hospital to start the induction process, I was 2 cm dilated on my own.

Between weeks 38 and 39, I did lots of squats and walking, we had sex a number of times (sorry, TMI!), I used red raspberry leaf and evening primrose oil supplements, and I also had an acupuncture session done to try to induce labor. I really think all of those things, combined with a strong core/pelvic floor from barre, meant that I was raring to go once we got to the hospital.

We were supposed to check in to Saint Joseph Regional Medical Center on Thursday, March 19th at 7 PM. What was happening at the hospital with our check-in and visitor policy was a moving target that week because of COVID19. I received a phone call in the afternoon letting me know that our check-in had been moved up to 5 PM! Seth rushed home from work, we had a decent dinner, and packed up our stuff.

On the way to the hospital, I started crying uncontrollably. I was pretty scared. Outside of when I was diagnosed with diabetes in 1992, and a bad bout with the flu during college, I had never been hospitalized. I also had never given birth! And I wasn't ready to be done being pregnant - it was my most favorite time of life, and we aren't guaranteed more children. Seth calmed me down, and in we went. We checked into room 4423 in labor and delivery, with Felissa as our night shift nurse.

When we got there, we got comfy, and they started some blood work and an IV line for me before we went over some paperwork about my medical conditions, preferences for baby, and food allergies. God bless Dr. Cavallo - he didn't order a diabetic diet for me, so I was able to choose the exact foods I wanted to eat. Much more on him later, but let's just say he is one of the best doctors I have ever known!

I had four very specific goals for my induction: 1. I wanted it to work. I knew an emergency C-section was always an option, but once we got started, I really didn't want to end up in surgery. 2. I wanted to wear my insulin pump and continuous glucose monitor throughout labor and be in control of my blood sugar. I wanted nothing to do with a glucose/insulin combo IV drip. 3. I did not want to have to use Pitocin. 4. I did not want to have an epidural. I'm a physical person, and I knew I wouldn't want to be tied to a bed if I didn't have to be.

At about 6:30 PM on Thursday night, Dr. Cavallo started something called a Cook catheter. It's a mechanical way to start labor induction. There are two balloons filled with saline that put pressure on the cervix from above and below to cause it to dilate and soften. Because I was already 2 cm dilated on my own, we were able to start there. I also started taking a pill called Cytotec in my cheek every two hours. This is also a "cervical ripener," and I would receive 8 doses by about 10:00 the next morning. At that point, we hunkered down for a long night.

I didn't really sleep much, between the medication doses, blood pressure, and blood sugar checks every two hours. Seth slept on the couch, though. I did have some decent contractions overnight, too, which were annoying, because I couldn't sleep through them, but I knew that they meant that the balloons were doing their job.

At the shift change the next morning, they drew more blood work, removed the balloons, and I got to meet our new nurse, Ashley, then I immediately asked if I could order breakfast! She said yes. She also checked me, and I was 4 cm dilated, which was progress, but we still had a long way to go. Ashley told me later that she didn't think we would have a baby during her shift!

A little while later, Dr. Sheikh came in to see me. I had consulted with Dr. Sheikh throughout my pregnancy for checks on me and specialized ultrasounds for the baby. He is the maternal fetal medicine doctor at St. Joe - it's his job to make sure that my pre-existing health conditions remain stable to keep me safe during pregnancy. What he told me next threw me for a loop - it appeared that I had developed mild preeclampsia. HUH!? My blood pressure had been perfect all throughout the pregnancy, and my urine tests in the office were never picking up protein. I noticed that my blood pressure was a little elevated since check-in, but I assumed it was because I was amped up. He said my creatinine levels from the night before were over the threshold to diagnose mild preeclampsia, and there was no longer any benefit to me or the baby to stay pregnant. I had to wait to eat until we had that morning's blood work and urine sample back. We would continue with the induction unless my blood work looked significantly worse. Then we might be talking about a C-section since I was only 4 cm.

Thankfully, about an hour later, we got word that my blood work looked better than the night before, and that, combined with a negative urine test, no headaches or blurry vision, and improved blood pressure readings, meant that I could eat breakfast and we would continue with the induction.

I had one more dose of Cytotec to get at about 10 AM, so in the meantime, Seth and I walked the halls. We were goofy, and super excited that it looked like we would meet our daughter that day! I got my last dose of medication and we tried to rest for a little bit. I asked Ashely to have Dr. Cavallo come talk to us about what was next in the induction process (Ashley had said that we would probably start Pitocin soon).

Dr. Cavallo stopped in at about 11 AM, and we discussed whether breaking my water or Pitocin was the right next step. He checked me, and I was 6 cm and 80% effaced! This was huge progress! He said if I were his wife, he would suggest we break my water before we introduce more medication, so that's what we did. And that's when EVERYTHING about my labor changed, very quickly!

Within minutes of breaking my water, my contractions got pretty strong. I had been warned that this would happen, but they still surprised me. We started playing "The Greatest Showman" soundtrack at this point to keep the mood light. Up next was "Hamilton," which was what was playing when our daughter was born!

Thankfully, our doula, Emily, was on her way, and Seth and I started practicing some of the things we had learned in our childbirth class, as well as things she had suggested during our meetings. Seth helped me breathe, in as un-panicked of a way as possible. He also advised me on my blood sugar. It was hanging out around 90, so I drank a little bit of apple juice. Closer to delivery, it crept up to about 140, which was higher than I would have liked, but still acceptable.

Ashley came back in to see me after noticing that I had gotten pretty.... vocal, pretty quickly. She checked me again, and within an hour of my water breaking, I was already 7 cm and 90% effaced. I'm pretty sure this is what they call "transition" in the stages of labor, and boy, did it get hard. Emily arrived then, too, and she and Seth helped me so much. I don't know how I would've handled each contraction without them!

Contractions at this stage are weird - there is so much pressure, and an intense need to push, but you can't do anything about it. I tried standing, sitting, dancing, and laying back down. I also started talking about an epidural at this point. I had had enough fluids that it would be possible in about 30 minutes if I really wanted one. But Ashley assured me that things were moving so quickly, if I could make it just a little while longer, we would be having my baby! Emily and Seth continued to keep me calm and breathing. Ashley checked me two more times in the next 30 minutes, and by the end of the 12:00 hour, I was "complete" and ready to push!

They got Dr. Cavallo, who was in a meeting about the Coronavirus. I found out later that he had actually called the meeting - I guess no one expected me to go from my water being broken to on the brink of delivery within less than two hours! I have to say, moving to the pushing stage of labor was a relief. Instead of just surviving through contractions, I could *actually do something! From this point forward was truly an out of body experience. I remember everything, but it doesn't feel like something that I actually did!*

Finally, Dr. Cavallo was ready for me. Everyone but me had a brief conversation about "Hamilton" and what a great show it is. I was vaguely aware of it. I do remember Seth remarking on my favorite line occurring very close to this point - when Aaron Burr is talking about having an affair with a British officer's wife, and Hamilton says "oh, shit!" I was mildly embarrassed that he outed me, but it did make me smile! I'm not sure how many contractions I pushed through with the doctor there at "go" time - I want to say 4, trying to get baby to move down that last little bit below my pelvis that she needed before being born. I asked him how I was doing, and he said each one was getting better. He called the pushes during my penultimate contraction "delivery pushes," which was what I needed to hear.

In the meantime, what I didn't know was that the baby's heart rate had been dipping during each contraction. Ashley quietly called NICU just in case they were needed.

Before the next contraction started, Dr. Cavallo told me that we were having a baby on my next contraction. Seth told me later that he could see something in my face shift upon hearing that. It started, and everyone started coaching me and cheering me on.

Three pushes later, and our daughter was born! The time was 1:35 PM. The umbilical cord was loosely around her neck, which Dr. Cavallo moved immediately. She was placed right on my chest, and Ashely rubbed her back to get her to take her first breath and then cry. That seemed like the longest time ever, especially since she was a little bit blue, but eventually she perked up after maybe 10 seconds, and NICU wasn't needed. I got to enjoy the next hour plus with her sweet face up by my face, marveling at the miracle we had created.

I'd love to say that that's where my labor and delivery story ends, but my uterus decided to go on strike at that point. Immediately after delivering the placenta (which looked healthy! Go me!), I started losing massive amounts of blood. The uterus is supposed to continue to contract after delivery to stop the blood supply that existed to the placenta. Mine had kicked it into high gear so quickly from 11:00 to 1:30 that it just tapped out and didn't do anything. Dr. Cavallo manually contracted it by pushing on my belly (which felt awesome…. heavy sarcasm), and they started Pitocin as well, but the meds that would also usually be used in this situation couldn't be used because of my blood pressure. I lost over a liter of blood, but thankfully I went into L&D with an abnormally high blood volume, so

I didn't need a transfusion. They started some IV pain meds for me at that point, too, as Dr. Cavallo continued to work on me to stop the bleeding. He remarked to me, "Oh, now you want pain meds!?" which made everyone giggle. I didn't stay on those for very long, though, because they made me feel really weird, loopy, and almost drunk. I had never had prescription pain meds before!

Finally, it seemed like the worst of the bleeding was done. Dr. Cavallo did some internal stitching to control other small cuts/tears, and we breastfed for the first time with help from a lactation consultant. Everyone got cleaned up, they weighed and measured her (a petite 6 lbs. 7 oz and 19 inches long), took her footprints and initial blood sugar, and we made our way to our mother and baby room, 4406. I was really lightheaded and woozy for the next few hours, so I was happy to be wheeled down the hall, helped to the bathroom, etc.

The last thing to note about L&D is the blood sugar checks they did on baby over the next twelve hours. Just after delivery, and first feeding they wanted her blood sugar above 45 - it was 69! We took 3 more readings before feedings, and they came in at 63, 89, and 56 - all above the threshold of 40 that had been set for her. Looking at her size and her blood sugar readings, no one would have known that her mama had type 1 diabetes. I could do a million amazing things every day for the rest of my life, and I will never be more proud of any one thing than I am about the fact that I nourished, grew, and birthed a perfect little baby whose health was not compromised because of my own shoddy immune system.

Was pregnancy with type 1 diabetes hard? YES. Was labor and delivery without pain meds hard? YES. But I achieved everything I wanted out of my pregnancy and labor process - a healthy, almost complication free pregnancy, a healthy baby, who was born after a successful, FAST induction, without an epidural or Pitocin, during which I wore my pump and CGM and controlled my own blood sugar, and with perfect blood sugars after birth. We have been on quite the journey to get this little one here, but I wouldn't trade it for anything. God's plan and timing is always perfect, and now I have my sweet Scarlett Alexandra to hold!

- Maggie Youngblood

My name is Rya. I have type 1 diabetes with supra-ventricular tachycardia and hypertension (non-diabetic related). Brief description of a long story: I've been diabetic for 5 plus years, and after being diagnosed, it took me a year to see that eating a standard diet didn't work for me. I knew that I needed to have a good A1C before getting pregnant, so I started working on getting back to healthy as soon as I switched my way of eating. I do not call it a diet; it's an entire way of being. Diets only last few weeks. As soon as the eating habits changed, the A1C went down to 5.5. I was at 5.1 when I got pregnant.

My glucose stayed well controlled the entire pregnancy. I'm on Omnipod and Dexcom. The technology was a lifesaver to me, I monitored the glucose on CGM, and made necessary adjustments on the insulin pump. In the first trimester, I did not have a lot of lows. It was easy to reduce the basal on the pump. The only lows I had was due to unexpected walking. We went to visit my parents and did some sightseeing. Sightseeing comes with a lot of walking. I didn't realize that. Also, my morning sickness got me from that point on. Hormones hit me hard. It was constant and lasted the entire day. Nothing worked until I asked for some meds. That solved that problem for me. See, vomiting gets complicated when you have type 1 diabetes. I didn't want to put myself at risk for dehydration.

I was tracking my basal increase weekly for my own reference. I was able to see the increase and decrease, etc. Basal requirements went up gradually until week 24; after that, it started going up a lot. During week 29, I had a considerable increase, and it stayed like that up until almost the end. It went down a little around week 36. My A1C at the end was 5.5.

The baby was growing and developing on schedule. Perinatologist visits would monitor the baby and measure everything. Now for a high-risk pregnancy, you have to go to a lot of doctors, and I mean a lot, but it's a good thing. I had my regular PCP monitoring my blood pressure, my OBGYN, perinatologist, endocrinologist, ophthalmologist, dentist. You have to stay on top of it all. It might sound overwhelming, but they are checking on your little bundle of joy that will not let you sleep for years. I think NSTs were my favorite with ultrasounds: you get to see your baby and hear that little heartbeat. I'm not crying; you're crying.

Now let me get back to that brief list of health conditions. My first non-diabetic pregnancy resulted in HELLP syndrome. My son was born healthy a few days short of being full term. Having HELLP syndrome puts you on another high-risk watch for pre-eclampsia. During my second pregnancy, I took pregnancy-approved blood pressure meds that worked great for the entire nine months. Few days before the scheduled induction, it started to go up. After some lab work, it was clear that we would be meeting our little girl a few days early.

My baby was born at 37 weeks 3 days at 6lbs and some ounces with normal blood sugar. No complications, no NICU. She stayed with me in the closet of my recovery room the entire time. My glucose was 70-120 the whole time. I kept a close eye on the Dexcom and made changes on the Omnipod. I was able to control my own glucose and keep my pump on; I just had to make sure it was out of the way. I gave both devices to my *husband to monitor while I was occupied with the baby delivering work. Nurses would come in periodically, ask me to prick my finger, and record the number. I was happy to oblige; it was helping me and helping them.*

Everybody was happy. As soon as the placenta was out, my glucose went back to normal and under. For a few days, my basal was only 3-4 units a day, a DAY! I know this is hard for me to envision too, but it was glorious. I was breastfeeding and pumping, so it took some playing around with basal/bolus to find what worked; after that, it was smooth sailing."
We stayed at the hospital for two days. As much as it was a wonderful experience, I was ready to get out of there and sleep those whole 30 minutes at home with the newborn. I am continuing my low carb journey. It is a way of life for me. I am determined to stay healthy without any diabetic complications by controlling my glucose and having normal numbers.

- Rya Bosley

When Things Don't Go as Planned

"I was at a large medical center's diabetes and pregnancy clinic. I was seen mostly by residents and fellows who were rude and knew little about Type 1 diabetes. The clinic's providers were rude and had a model of scaring patients about the risks of hyperglycemia, and then acting surprised when (due to the fear they reinforce all the time) patients strive for lower than recommended blood sugars. It was disempowering, and I was treated like I was nothing more than Type 1 diabetes - never a woman who was excited and nervous to be pregnant and who also happened to have Type 1. The labor was not great - the hospital would not let me wear my pump and they could not manage the IV drip well. There were all kinds of medical students and endocrinology fellows who did not contribute anything to the process.

Afterwards I had terrible yeast mastitis - so painful and a midwife there told me that she wouldn't treat me because she recently read an article that it may not be real. I was so overwhelmed with everything and the lack of support. I even told one of the providers at my follow up that I thought I may have postpartum depression. She told me that everyone got "the blues," and that I'd be fine with no further follow up or questions."

-Anjali Asrani

Sometimes for all the planning we make, things don't go the way we want them to, and this can be very difficult as childbirth is something many of us dreamed about since we were little children. If things don't go as planned, give yourself time to heal. Don't beat yourself up for feeling bad even though you ended up with a healthy baby.

Mourn your birth experience if you need to. I was depressed for 5 years after my second cesarean. Being able to VBAC my last baby was a very healing experience that I am so grateful for, but not everyone is so lucky.

When I had arrived at the hospital around 10:30 pm, we already had agreed upon my birth plan (the OBs who ultimately made the calls as well as the midwives, who had jointly had a meeting to discuss my case). That included among other things that I would manage my own blood sugar and that I would have intermittent monitoring (unless there was an indication that we needed to do continuous monitoring). When I arrived at the hospital they were swamped and there were no rooms available. When one did finally open up, I had a postpartum nurse attending to me (and not a very good one), due to the fact that the L&D nurses were all busy with other moms. We handed over my insulin pens (I do MDI), and the nurse was supposed to bring the insulin to the pharmacy to get approval and bring them back so I could use them.

For several hours, I was left alone in the room and the nurse didn't come by and never brought me my insulin back. I did have an extra rapid acting insulin pen with me, but I was unable to take my basal dose at the right time. This did, ultimately, make my blood sugars rise a little higher than I was comfortable with. I didn't end up getting approval for my pens until late the following morning.

Additionally, around 7AM there was a shift change and the midwife that came on duty delivered me an ultimatum: If I was going to have her deliver my baby, I had to go on continuous monitoring. Otherwise, I would have to be under the OB's care. I showed her my birth plan that clearly stated that I would have intermittent monitoring and there was even the signature of the OB next to it. She didn't care. And unfortunately, since the wireless monitors had been recalled just a week or so prior, I was stuck with the wired monitor. That meant that I couldn't move more than a foot or two beyond the hospital bed, nor could I go to the bathroom, use the shower, etc. The continuous monitoring really slowed down my contractions.

I desperately wanted to give birth with the help of the midwives, not the OBs, so I just went along with this and requested as many bathroom breaks as I could get. Unlike the previous night where I was left mostly alone, now I had a student in the room at all times and nurses and midwives were coming in frequently. They no longer granted me permission to inject myself insulin because my blood sugar went to 120 and I had written in my birth plan that I wanted to maintain blood sugar between 70 and 120 (nowhere did I state that the hospital would take

*over if I went beyond that, but that's how they decided to pursue this).
Due to missing my basal dose at the appropriate time, my blood sugar had
steadily risen. At one point after their 'takeover' I was having some food
and the nurse made a call to the OB to ask what my insulin dose should
be. I told her the Insulin to carb ratio, and she ignored that (even though
it was written plainly on my birth plan with the signature of my CDE).
Instead, the dose they provided was probably half what it was supposed to
be and of course, it didn't help my blood sugar at all.*

*My blood sugar rose to 180. At that point, I requested to 'please let me
manage my own blood sugar, as I know what I am doing!' Their response
was that I was now too close to give birth and just let it go. I did end up
giving birth within 30-40 minutes. Fortunately, despite a prolonged labor
and pushing, the baby never showed any signs of distress.*

-Amelia Kissick

Advocate for yourself. Make your wishes clear before your birth and if your
doctor doesn't agree, find a new one! I made sure that my doctor would allow
me to keep my pump and cgm and to handle diabetes management myself
after my bad experience with my second baby. Ask lots of questions. Will they
confiscate your insulin?

Require an insulin drip? Only give you a limited amount of time to deliver
vaginally? Will they whisk the baby away right after birth even if the baby is
healthy? Think about all the possibilities and make a plan. Obviously, plans
don't always work out, but preparing and making sure your wishes line up with
the doctor's and the hospital guidelines will be immensely helpful.

Chapter 17: 40 Weeks and Beyond

Going Past Your Due Date

Going past 40 weeks is not common in type 1 diabetic mamas. There are a few doctors who will allow it if control is *very* tight. My MFM doctor had given me permission to go to 41 weeks, but I was scared by the estimated weight (which was totally wrong!) I have seen a few very dedicated mamas do it, so if it's something you and your doctor are comfortable with, go for it! You'll definitely want increased monitoring though.

Postpartum

As previously mentioned, you'll see a pretty drastic drop in insulin needs postpartum, even more so if you're

breast-feeding. I found that this could not be remedied by adjusting basal insulin as it was unpredictable and just had to keep glucose nearby when nursing.

After the initial few weeks of lows, many moms start seeing insulin needs increase and struggle more. It can be a very difficult time as you are sleep-deprived, focused on baby, and now that you aren't pregnant, you probably aren't as focused on your numbers. Don't give up just because your baby has been born! With postpartum depression being a possibility, high blood sugars will increase that risk. When blood glucose is high, we urinate out the nutrients needed to make neurotransmitters in the brain and depression is more likely. Normal blood sugars will also help in recovery from both a vaginal delivery and a c-section.

Postpartum Bleeding

Postpartum bleeding and discharge (lochia) can last from a few days to 6 weeks. You will have this whether you delivered vaginally or by cesarean. The bleeding may be lighter if you have a cesarean because the doctor may use suction to "clean" your uterus out, but don't count on this.

The bleeding will be bright red for the first 3 days or so and you may have clots. The clots should not be bigger than a quarter. The bleeding should become lighter after around 10 days. The color will go from red to pink to brown, to yellowish white at the end.

You don't want to use tampons during this time as they could cause an infection. I liked Always Infinity pads, but many mamas swear by Depends (disposable undergarments) during this time.

Breastfeeding

There is absolutely NO reason that you can't breastfeed if you so choose. I've had many t1 mamas tell me that they were told they couldn't nurse because of diabetes, and nothing can be further from the truth. Nursing your baby might even help prevent them from developing t1 in the future.

Some ask if diabetes causes milk supply issues and I am not aware of any reason that it should, but there is some evidence that insulin resistance can lead to low milk supply. Metformin has shown to be helpful with this. The biggest piece of advice I can give you for nursing is not to supplement formula. AT ALL. I had many well-meaning people tell me, "let Daddy feed the baby" or "give yourself a break, one bottle won't hurt", but it did hurt. I was never able to get the same amount of milk pumping and my supply dwindled. This was an exceedingly frustrating experience that caused such heartache. I felt like I was starving my baby and ended up feeding my first two babies formula due to low milk supply. With number 3, I didn't supplement once, other than for one week while I was taking a strong medication that could have hurt the baby, so I gave him a homemade organic formula and religiously pumped. I had no supply issues with him. My supply was overabundant actually, despite eating less than 30g of carbohydrate per day.

Another piece of advice, or knowledge really; you'll hear people tell you that if it hurts, you aren't doing it right. I'm going to tell you, nursing HURTS. My nipples bled with my first. It took a good two weeks before nursing became comfortable. It didn't come naturally to me, and don't feel bad if it doesn't come naturally to you. I had to be taught how to get my baby to latch correctly. Take advantage of the lactation consultants and don't be embarrassed to ask for help. Use the help line if it's offered. Make sure you're using cream on your nipples. Cooling packs can help with the pain of engorgement and make sure to have lots of nursing pads as you will definitely leak in the early days. I've also had questions about whether high blood sugars affect your milk. Most doctors will tell you no, but in my experience it absolutely does. I'm always doing experiments and while I was nursing my last baby, I frequently tested my milk on my glucose meter. I've also seen that babies of mamas with high blood sugars tend to gain more weight. This is just my observance.

If my blood sugar was high, I didn't see it reflected in the milk right away, but I did hours later. I chose to pump and dump after running high.

I also found that eating low carb lowered the amount of glucose in my milk. This is completely anecdotal, but I had a few other t1 mamas check their milk and the non-low-carb ones read much higher than mine (400's vs 20's and 30's). The literature is very much lacking on this topic and everything I've read says that carbohydrate content of mother's milk stays the same regardless of diet, but my little experiments say otherwise. I'm aware that the meter tests glucose rather than lactose, but the rise in glucose makes me think there is something to it.

In the first few weeks, you'll likely experience lows when breastfeeding. Make sure to always have hypo treatments available when you are nursing your baby. No basal adjustment I tried worked to avoid this, but this balances out after a few weeks.

Losing the Baby Weight

I gained about the same amount of weight with all of my babies; around 30lb. With my first two standard-diet pregnancies, the baby weight took years to come off. I was still carrying the weight from baby #2, four years later. As soon as I lost the weight, I became pregnant of course!

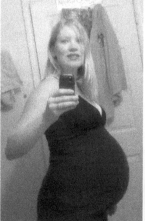 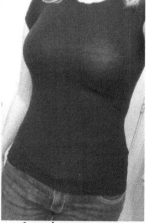

The morning of my induction   **4 weeks postpartum**

After my low carb pregnancy, the weight basically came off immediately. When I left the hospital, you could not even tell I had been pregnant. I was wearing a size small t-shirt. The weight just fell off. It was an unbelievable difference.

You Can Do This!

A type 1 pregnancy can be a very stressful thing, but with normal blood sugars using Dr Bernstein's protocols, it can be a *LOT* less stressful with fewer highs and lows. My Grit mamas have a much easier time, with the majority having full-term, complication-free pregnancies with normal weight babies. It's not easy by any means, but it is worth it when you hold that little bundle of joy in your arms. I continued eating low-carb and still do to this day (11 years later). It is absolutely sustainable in the long term, and I'm healthier than ever thanks to Dr. Bernstein.

Recommended Reading

Dr. Bernstein's Diabetes Solution. Richard K. Bernstein, MD

Balancing Pregnancy with Pre-Existing Diabetes: Healthy Mom, Healthy Baby. Cheryl Alkon

Managing Your Gestational Diabetes. Lois Jovanovic-Peterson, MD

Pregnancy with Type 1 Diabetes. Ginger Vieira, CPT & Jennifer C. Smith, RD, CDCES

Real Food for Gestational Diabetes. Lily Nichols, RDN, CDCES

Stop the Thyroid Madness. Janie A. Bowthorpe, M.Ed.

Taking Charge of Your Fertility. Toni Weschler, MPH

The Low Carb Dietitian's Guide to Health and Beauty. Franziska Spritzler, RD, CDCES

Lightning Source UK Ltd.
Milton Keynes UK
UKHW011905010222
398052UK00001B/201